1991

Medical Staff Peer Review

A Strategy for Motivation and Performance

Daniel A. Lang, M.D.

AHA books are published by
American Hospital Publishing, Inc.,
an American Hospital Association company

Library of Congress Cataloging-in-Publication Data

Lang, Daniel A.
  Medical staff peer review : a strategy for motivation and performance / Daniel A. Lang.
        p.   cm.
  Includes bibliographical references.
  ISBN 1-55648-065-2
  1. Hospitals—medical staff—Evaluation. 2. Peer review.
I. Title.
  [DNLM: 1. Medical Staff. 2. Motivation. 3. Peer Review—methods. W 84 L269m]
  RA972.L27   1991
  362.1'1'0683—dc20
  DNLM/DLC
  for Library of Congress   90-14532
                                                                 CIP

Catalog no. 145157

©1991 by American Hospital Publishing, Inc.,
an American Hospital Association company

Printed in the USA

AHA is a service mark of the American Hospital Association used under license by American Hospital Publishing, Inc.

Text set in Palatino
3M—03/91—0291

Audrey Kaufman, Project Editor
Linda Conheady, Manuscript Editor
Marcia Bottoms, Managing Editor
Peggy DuMais, Production Coordinator
Marcia Vecchione, Designer
Brian Schenk, Books Division Director

To Charlotte, who has no peers,
and Leonard and Doris, who outrank us all.

Contents

List of Figures and Tables

Figures

Figures

Tables

About the Author

Daniel A. Lang, M.D., is the medical director of the National Health Foundation in Los Angeles. He is responsible for the professional education program of the foundation, which is an affiliate of the Hospital Council of Southern California. As the only physician affiliated with a metropolitan council on a full-time basis, Dr. Lang provides assistance to medical staffs and boards in achieving individual and joint goals.

Currently, Dr. Lang writes and edits a newsletter for medical staff officers entitled *The Medical Executive Committee Reporter.* He has also written a book entitled *The Disabled Physician: Problem-Solving Strategies for the Medical Staff,* published by American Hospital Publishing, 1989. Dr. Lang teaches a six-session graduate-style seminar for physician leaders that covers the operational aspects of medical staff management. He is a recognized expert on hospital–medical staff relations in southern California.

Dr. Lang is a board-certified internist who, after 20 years of private practice, served as medical director of Brotman Medical Center (a 500-bed tertiary community hospital in Culver City, California). He is a clinical assistant professor of medicine at UCLA Medical Center. In addition, Dr. Lang is active in organized medicine and is the past president of the Bay District of the Los Angeles County Medical Association and a member of the editorial board of that society. He has also served as the medical director and vice-president of Area XXII PSRO.

Acknowledgments

Special thanks are extended to Patricia Perfetti, who rendered yeoman services in the preparation of this manuscript. Dr. J. Raymond Hinshaw and June N. Lang provided editorial review and reality testing.

Financial support for this project was furnished by the National Health Foundation.

Introduction:
The Legitimacy of Peer Review

Medical staffs are the focus of rising controversy. As hospitals invest in screening systems for the evaluation of patient care, medical staffs are confronted with information, previously unavailable, about physician performance. Whereas in the "preinformation era" occasional cases were identified by catastrophe or jungle drums, now, as a consequence of concurrent and retrospective review of all clinical services, the number of cases for physician review has risen dramatically. Each month the medical staff is presented with a range of problems, from minor policy deviations to major clinical performance failures. In addition to individual cases, modern data processing allows for trend development—by physician, by service, hospitalwide, and by diagnosis. Inferences, if not judgments, about effectiveness and efficiency of care are now within reach of the medical staff. This information flow creates an opportunity to monitor care and strive for its continuing improvement.

A parallel development has been the acceptance that the medical staff of the acute care hospital has the authority to evaluate its members. That authority comes via federal and state law, through the governing body of the hospital. It comes as well from professional tradition, though this is mistrusted by the general authorities. Authority also arises from public expectation. Here the trust is even less and the authority is under constant review to ensure the fairness of its application. Authority also comes from the physician membership who through their bylaws create the structures and functions in which it is vested.

The combination of opportunity and authority creates an obligation on the part of the medical staff to evaluate the performance of its members in the interest of self-improvement. The obligation flows in many directions—to the patient in the effort to ensure quality (or truth in marketing); to the governing body in support of that entity's need to assure the public of the effectiveness of the hospital's peer review; to its members to create a professionally secure environment for clinical practice; to licensure and accreditation authorities that seek to protect the patient, the hospital, and its physicians by the promulgation and enforcement of standards; and to the general public at large, which anxiously seeks assurance of the adequacy and effectiveness of its health services.

Widespread recognition of the obligation and, indeed, growing penalties for the failure to take it seriously have led to increased support for medical staff self-improvement efforts. Hospital investment in screening systems is the first step. It is easiest to allocate specific funds to acquire hardware, software, and personnel to produce data. Harder is the enlistment of physician expertise in the design of screening and data systems, but here the marketplace has stepped in to fill the gap. More difficult still is the enlistment, organization, and instruction of physicians to convert the data into information that is useful in judging physician and hospital services. Part of that difficulty comes from the recognition that somewhere at the end of the process lies the need to confront performance failure and to take effective corrective action. The seriousness of this last step is not lost on physicians, nor should it be.

Recognition of the ultimate step has led to the support of the intervening ones. Hospitals have invested in education and training in medical staff management for physicians. Chiefs of staff are often compensated for the very real time expended on medical staff administration. There is a growing pool of trained physician executives whose principal raison d'etre is the oversight and management of quality assurance and peer review activities. The result has been an enhanced capability of medical staffs to carry out the obligations listed above.

Four elements, then, create the legitimacy of the peer review process—opportunity, authority, obligation, and capability. Each is essential in the development of an effective system in which physicians entrust their futures to the review of their fellows. Failure of the hospital to recognize and foster these elements is incompatible with institutional life.

These elements are generic with features that are common across hospitals and state lines. However, each hospital also has unique features. Medical staffs will be more or less structured and their members will vary in their faith in the democratic process and in their skill to operate within the complex human organization that is the modern hospital. Governing bodies will seek more or less control, have various amounts of money, and be subject to varying degrees of public or private limitations. Governments and regulators will differ in their faith in the institution's professional self-regulation over inspection and punishment—all in the name of patient protection.

There is doubt that the organized medical staff of the acute care hospital is up to the job of professional regulation. Pressures to shift the authority to state licensing, federal and state reimbursement agencies, and private contractors have become almost relentless. The press daily charts rising governmental and public concern over the effectiveness and, hence, trustworthiness of the peer review process. This mistrust spills over to physicians, exacerbating their concern for the fairness of the manner in which they will be judged.

The organized medical staff must earn the right to judge and rule its members. Just as there is no divine right of succession, there is no God-given irrevocable mandate for medical staffs to determine the fates of their members. Just as the right to self-review must be earned from outside the profession, so also must physicians be willing to participate in and submit to the judgment and rule of their colleagues. That willingness is not automatically bestowed by a signature on the bottom of an application or a letter of appointment. It is implanted and nurtured by fair and effective medical staff processes. It achieves full growth with realization by physicians that they have ownership interest in the medical staff. It comes from physicians' recognition that they get something back from membership. A physician is always sitting in judgment of the degree to which the medical staff meets his or her expectations. Success in meeting physician expectations, then, is usually accompanied by participation in physician rule.

This book provides tools and strategies for the performance of effective peer review. The text presents an analysis of the peer review process and its component steps; an approach to the enlistment of physician support in the peer review process; a review of the roles of the governing body and the Medical Executive Committee, which are central to the creation of the values that foster effective peer review; an overview of the current legal issues; a system for self-evaluation; and, in the appendix, test scenarios to help clarify applications of principles to practical situations. Serious consideration of the principles as set forth in this book will help foster the effective performance of medical staff peer review.

The Peer Review Crisis

Peer review is in trouble. The very concept of physician reviewing physician is under serious challenge. The efficacy of collegial review in the assurance of quality care or public safety has been called into question. Despite authority for peer review in statutes and professional codes, patients, payers, government regulators, and even other physicians have come to challenge this hallowed practice. Objectivity, fairness, and efficiency have all been doubted by participants in, or beneficiaries of, the process. Alternatives to peer review by the organized medical staff are being actively promoted, both in and out of government.

□ Causes of Peer Review Mistrust

Physician mistrust of peer review starts with the organized medical staff. Its traditional collegial approach to problem solving is inadequate to cope with the economic and legal implications of physician privilege determinations. Despite a growing need for collective or group consciousness, competition and uncertainty have made many physicians less trusting of their peers. Even a small medical staff may be unable to maintain the legendary collegiality. Somehow the senior arm around the junior shoulder, accompanied by the fatherly words, "We don't do that here—let me show you a better way," is a vanishing phenomenon. Those words would be challenged as lacking objectivity and documentation, let alone purity of motivation. A member of a small medical staff of a rural hospital recently complained to me, "The friendly days are gone. In medical staff meetings, we can't refer to doctors by name. We have to use numbers."

Mistrust of the organized medical staff may be well-founded. The Joint Commission on Accreditation of Healthcare Organizations (JCAHO), the "physician's own" accrediting body, has found monitoring and evaluation of patient care by the medical staff to be the most common deficiency in the survey process. Lack of effective corrective action is equally common. Simply translated, the medical staff does not always exhibit a firm commitment to the identification of substandard care or to the improvement of physician performance. Where the medical staff seeks to effect change, it is often without the support of objective standards or well-defined processes. Motivation for action is not always clear or based on a concern for quality.

The mistrust arises from a number of factors, not the least of which has been the manner in which care has been reviewed. Random, subjective, superficial analysis has been found wanting both by those performing the activity and by those benefiting from its laxity. No wonder, then, that the recipient of medical staff attention may feel unfairly singled out. Even the physician associated with a professional performance failure can point to the evident or perceived inequity. Underlying the rationalization or the protest is the complaint, often valid, that others committed the same errors and somehow escaped detection. Against that background, almost any medical staff action might appear unfair or biased. Therefore, other physicians could justify their natural unwillingness to participate in judging their peers with the comment "It's a witch-hunt" or "There but for the grace of Providence go I."

The uneven nature of the process of peer review fosters other beliefs. Physicians with departmental or medical staff political power, by manipulating the peer review process, can derail the career of a less-fortunate competitor. *Patrick v. Burget*[1] illustrates that kind of conflict. In this case, a physician successfully claimed that members of his department deprived him of his privileges for economic motives. The range of matters over which physicians can compete unfairly is broad, indeed. Prominence in the joint hospital–medical staff geographic franchise or marketplace is perhaps the most common. Economic dominance is usually the goal but power, authority, and stature may be others. Scientific dispute may also lead to peer review conflict. Given the uncertain basis for some medical staff procedures or their various indications, there is ample room for dispute that may be carried to extreme by an assault by one physician on the medical staff privileges of another. It is not inconceivable that one surgeon might address a rival for the affections of the operating room supervisor through the vehicle of medical staff peer review.

Even supporters of peer review lose heart over questions of efficiency or efficacy. In the abstract, most would regard it a plus that the individual physician is protected from arbitrary and capricious action by medical staff authorities. Yet, just as in other areas of jurisprudence in our society, an inordinately long time may elapse between the detection of an inappropriate act and the sequence of restraint, adjudication, limitation, and appeal. While this lengthy process wends its cautious way, the physician may continue with practice rights undisturbed. Society is losing patience with this dilatory pace. On the other hand, the price of premature or inappropriate imposition of restraints or limits is high. Summary suspension of clinical or professional rights and privileges is even more hazardous.

Of more concern than the slowness of peer review is the uncertain result. Protections in medical staff bylaws and oversight by the courts often have allowed the guilty to go free. Again, this is a hallowed expression of a basic American concern for individual liberty. But the physician who is a voluntary participant in the judgment or limitation of his or her peers is likely to resent the interference of outsiders when a decision is finally made to take action against a colleague. This tends to further diminish the support of the peer reviewer for the work. If a judgment is reversed, it may be difficult to get the peer reviewer to volunteer next time, regardless of commitment to the underlying concept.

Voluntary participation in peer review is lessened by the efforts of society to address these issues. Within the medical staff structure are procedural safeguards that appropriately limit arbitrary action. As a result, peer review now must be more painstaking and laborious. Objective screening and statistical data bases, developed to make physician review more objective and automatic, generate more work rather than less. The reviewer must learn new techniques that supplement or even challenge intuitive professional skills. Regardless of fairness and skill, within the hospital community is a political and professional backwash that may drown the reviewer. Participation in peer review in the acute care general hospital is an act of uncommon social responsibility and political courage.

It is an act of legal bravery as well. Internal process safeguards, established to make peer review fair, create a minefield in which even the most wary may stumble. The reviewer may be literally destroyed in the ensuing explosion. The allegation that the reviewer is biased, unfair, anticompetitive, racially motivated, or merely unskilled in following the rules imposes a burden of defense, not within the relative protection of the medical staff bylaws but in the cold harsh light of state and federal court. It is sufficient to allege anticompetitive motivation and to assert an effect on interstate commerce (*Pinhas v. Summit Health, Ltd.*)[2] to shift the venue to the federal court. The medical staff structure, with its focus on the protection of quality by the evaluation of care rendered, is bypassed. The issue becomes unfair trade practices. It is ironic that by encouraging this shift, the federal court is saying that the protection of quality is secondary to that of fair economic competition. So long as businesses compete, even in the manufacture of bad products or less-than-useful services, one branch of the federal government apparently is willing to cast a blind eye.

One can interpret the court's willingness to preempt the organized medical staff as indicative of the attitude that peer review in the acute care hospital is not legitimate. It may not observe the niceties of process so dear to legal minds and therefore can be rejected on its face. In the minds of some, that rejection is not to be grieved over, because medical staffs are thought to be reluctant to take action even if processes are followed. When action is taken it is apt to be oblique and diffident. Worse, it is unlikely to have a significant impact on the quality of care. Given that, why not punish the reviewer for working under "false pretenses"?

Payers decry the weakness of peer review in the struggle for cost containment. This is especially frustrating in the acute care general hospital setting. Peer review here achieves its legitimacy in the protection of the quality of care. Actions against physicians who waste resources or otherwise fail to practice efficiently can be sustained only if a nexus with quality can be shown. Paradoxically, therefore, peer review in the acute care general hospital may only serve to increase costs, at least in the context of a specific case. Shortsightedly, payers seek to pay for care at a rate that is insufficient to support effective medical staff review. Hospitals spend less than 0.5 percent of total sales on peer review and quality assurance. In other industries, 2 to 5 percent is the norm. This is an expression of an attitude on the part of some hospital managers that because of low profit margins, the hospital cannot afford to upgrade or defend its quality with expensive, and perhaps ineffective, peer review.

The patient may not see the connection between peer review and the protection of the general public. One could argue—and attorneys do—that the rise in professional liability suits in the past 15 years is an appropriate societal mechanism for the control of quality because professional peer review has failed. The professional "conspiracy of silence" that allows poor care to continue without medical protest or restraint is frequently alleged. These events only serve to reinforce the general societal distrust of professional authority systems. They are perceived as defending the monopoly of its membership, to the detriment of the general welfare.

Even members of related professions decry the deficiencies of the peer review process. In the acute care hospital, "nurses get fired while doctors get letters" is the common complaint when both professions are involved in the same clinical performance failure. Whereas this overstatement ignores the very real protections that salaried hospital professionals enjoy and the rising number of physicians whose clinical privileges are limited or eliminated, nonetheless there is a general skepticism that peer review is not hard enough on bad docs. The protection it affords is limited and, in the view of some, perhaps not worth the bother.

This attitude and, therefore, concern about the legitimacy of great investment in peer review at a time of cost constraints has reached official expression. One may interpret the conflict between the JCAHO and the New York State Health Department as a paradigm for an assault on the effectiveness of professional peer review as a guardian of standards and quality.[3] The JCAHO is an embodiment of the view that voluntary professional standards, monitored and enforced by the voluntary action of peers, are more effective in improving the quality of patient care. The health department espouses the view that quality is better guarded by standards set in law, monitored by police authority, and enforced by civil and criminal penalties. This dichotomy is the health care expression of the fundamental Manichaean dispute about the inherent goodness or evil of man. So far, it seems the seers of evil are in the ascendancy.

The federal government has also sided with the critics of the medical staff. Medicare beneficiaries are safeguarded through the oversight of a professional review organization (PRO) that operates in nearly total independence from the medical staff. Regardless of the effectiveness of the hospital's own review body, the PRO cannot yield any authority but must perform its own quality evaluations and take its own corrective actions against physicians. In doing so it sets a pattern for external review. Although PROs are considered by some as a "peer review organization," this is so only in a broad generic sense. The role of the PRO is regulatory. It undercuts the authority and influence of the organized medical staff and in the long run is a threat to its existence.

☐ Making Peer Review Legitimate

If professional peer review is to prevail at the hospital level, it must reassert its legitimacy in ways that restore its prior support. However, it may be too late to achieve this end because of the strength of its adversaries. Indeed, it may seek a status quo ante that never was except in theory. Nonetheless, if the heart of a profession is self-regulation through monitoring of voluntarily set standards, medical staffs cannot escape the challenge to make peer review work.

First, physicians must become passionate partisans for the concept. The willingness to participate in and abide by the judgment of peers is the sine qua non of the subculture that is the organized medical staff. Peer review is valued only if membership in that subculture is valued. Membership, therefore, must convey unique benefits to make submission to the peer review process worthwhile.

Second, the relationship between the judgment of peers and the protection of the patient must be made explicit. Professional judgment alone will not restore peer review to a level of confidence. Only by convincing others that society, not just doctors, is protected by peer review will it be possible to minimize the intrusion of agencies seeking to wrest control away from the profession. Ours is a society that holds that you can't trust the objectivity of experts. Only a clear demonstration that peer review is essential for public health can reverse this perception.

Paradoxically, because of the risk of lawsuits, the rising complexity of the medical staff quasi-judicial process, and the need to spend professional time to earn a living in an era of cost containment, physicians may be unwilling to commit to effective peer review. Absent that commitment there can be no legitimacy, only regulation, penalty, and restraint. Medical staffs have within reach a system for the provision of peer review in a manner that can be supported by physicians and the public at large. Whether it will be in the long run is very much up to the physicians themselves.

□ *References*

1. Patrick v. Burget, 846, U.S. 94 (1988).
2. Pinhas v. Summit Health, Ltd., 880, F.2d 1108 (9th Cir. 1989).
3. Physicians hide problems when "peer review is under siege." *Hospital Peer Review* 14(7):81–84, July 1989.

□ *Additional Reading*

Blum, J. D. Medical peer review. *Journal of Legal Education,* pp. 525–33, 1988 [no further information available].

Furrow, B. R. Peer review: teaching the relation of cost and quality. *Journal of Legal Education,* pp. 535–44, 1988 [no further information available].

Muller, F. H. Teaching health law students. *Journal of Legal Education,* pp. 545–54, 1988 [no further information available].

Schwartz, W. B., and Mendelson, D. N. The role of physician-owned insurance companies in the detection and deterrence of negligence. *Journal of the American Medical Association* 262(10):1335–41, Sept. 8, 1989.

Peer Review:
The Essence of the Professional

At the core, the physician believes he or she is without peers. Despite that, through socialization and acculturation physicians are expected to exhibit certain common characteristics in response patterns. With more professional training those patterns acquire narrower limits of appropriateness and higher standards of competency. Specialty training sharpens the perspective further. At each level, the number of individuals who could call themselves peers decreases. For the most specialized activities, only a relative few can claim peer status. More common professional and nonprofessional activities are shared by larger groups. This chapter explores the concept and definition of a *peer* and outlines the five components of an effective peer review system.

□ Definition of a Peer

The concept of the peer, then, is activity-specific. A highly trained neurosurgeon skilled in stereotactic and laser surgery of the interior of the brain is indeed uniquely specialized, and evaluation of his technique must be by someone similarly trained. But the indication for the surgery and the functional outcome of the patient are within the competence and scope of practice of the clinical neurologist who lacks the manual skill. The knowledge of general medicine, adherence to medical staff rules and regulations, and general professional demeanor are even less specific and, hence, capable of effective review by the medical staff as a whole. Activities outside the organized medical staff, reflecting adherence to ordinary standards of civil behavior, may be judged by an even broader social group.

This obvious hierarchy of peer authority is an important concept often challenged by physicians undergoing review. Although fairness and accuracy require that action based on specialty performance be evaluated by those at that skill level, it does not follow that all actions of a specialist require such high-level assessment; nor are the consequences of specialty failure solely within the purview of that small group of experts.

To illustrate, consider an inappropriate death in surgery associated with a specialty procedure. The initial general screening mechanisms of the medical staff would identify the case for review. A nonspecialist might participate in the decision to refer for specialty review. Specialists would determine that the death was inappropriate and avoidable and therefore the basis for some corrective response. The nature of that response, if significant, would be determined by the broadly based medical staff. Whereas the specialist is required to identify the specific act of omission or commission, the medical staff must respond to the broader issue of inappropriate death due to technical failure. The latter transgression is capable of being characterized generically and therefore is within the purview of the broader-based body.

The issue might become even more generic if fundamental competence as a physician is involved or there is the possibility of civil negligence or a criminal act. In these instances, the review process becomes still broader, involving societal mechanisms such as the courts or administrative boards. The peer group here includes nonprofessionals because the act committed was a breach of broader significance than mere specialized technical failure.

☐ Techniques of Peer Review

Review of physician performance occurs in a hierarchical way conducted by differing entities for different purposes. Review involves the screening of all care rendered against a group of indicators that are accepted by the medical staff as flags for the identification of cases that might reflect substandard management. These indicators are, of necessity, broad and generic. Information is obtained from this generic screening process in two ways: Individual cases are subjected to analysis to disclose the presence and the nature of the professional performance failure as a basis for possible corrective action related to the single event. Information is gleaned as well from the aggregation of experience into a composite and longitudinal picture of a physician's clinical activity.

Peer review, then, uses different techniques in achieving its goals. The time-hallowed way involves the in-depth review of the exceptional case, searching for preventable causes of untoward events. Some critics would hold that the search is really for justification of such events by the identification of factors beyond professional control. This will be considered in detail subsequently. With modern data processing, it has become more convenient to develop rate and trend information that is also indicative. The frequency with which a procedure is performed, if low, may signal increased risk to patients.[1] Next may be the collection of exceptions such as the frequency of a particular complication or an unanticipated and preventable death. A more specific set of measures looks at certain aspects of care, comparing them against the physician's own historical performance, as well as that of various local and national peer groups. Thus, if one monitors the time required to perform an emergency Cesarean section from the time the anesthesiologist says "cut" to the time the infant is delivered, one can determine whether a single case took too long, whether a particular surgeon has a pattern of being slow, or whether over time, the surgeon's performance has slowed. Each of these measures may impart different information and require different analysis and, ultimately, distinctive corrective action.

An effective peer review system has five components:

- *Direct concurrent observation of physician performance.* Direct observation in which communication skills, analytic ability, professional knowledge, and manual capability are assessed is part of the process of evaluation of the new medical staff member. It is also used to investigate a physician who has experienced a clinical performance failure.
- *A screening system in which all care is reviewed against outcome and process standards developed by the medical staff.* This screening, for the sake of cost and efficiency, usually is not done by physicians, although it is the work of and for physicians and is therefore part of the peer review process. Physicians challenge screening on the grounds that it represents the hospital's administrative intrusion into the peer review process. When this process is properly operated, the hospital merely supplies the personnel and support systems; the physicians own the screening indicators and the information that comes out of the process.
- *A first-level exception analysis by physicians of cases that fail screening.* First-level review validates the screening failure. This review may attempt to assign individual responsibility and to characterize more precisely the performance failure. Ultimately the reviewer is responsible for making the departmental referral decision. First-level review need not be precisely specialized.
- *Definitive exception analysis at the clinical department level.* The goal here is for specialists to provide professional analysis of the events in the case. The definitive exception responsibility is to present this analysis in terms understandable to nonspecialists, in sufficient detail to support the validity of the specialty conclusion.

- *Aggregation of individual events into a composite picture.* These events reflect patterns and trends that provide a background for the understanding of the exceptional case. The ultimate goal of the physician-performance profile is to identify declining skills before egregious clinical failure occurs.

These five elements of peer review must occur in a broader context. In the acute care hospital or the large medical group, that context is the organized medical staff. Effective peer review cannot take place in the absence of an organized medical staff. In turn, the raison d'etre of the medical staff is meaningful, thoughtful peer review.

□ *Reference*

1. Hannan, E. L., and others. Investigation of the relationship between volume and mortality for surgical procedures performed in New York State hospitals. *Journal of the American Medical Association* 262(4):503–510, July 28, 1989.

☐ Chapter 3

The Process of Direct Peer Review

Peer review encompasses two fundamental activities: evaluation of performance by direct observation and analysis of the record of performance. These two activities are complementary. Each has a distinct place, and each has unique limitations. The role of the medical staff is to provide for both of these functions in the proper mix to ensure the effective and efficient assessment of the work of physicians. This chapter discusses performance evaluation by direct peer observation—the various opportunities for such observation and its inherent limitations.

☐ Opportunities for Direct Observation

The organized medical staff has four opportunities to exercise concurrent and direct observation in assessing physician performance without a prior formal judgment that a given case requires special review. These opportunities occur during the intake interview, provisional monitoring or proctoring, consultation, and investigational monitoring.

The Intake Interview

On application for medical staff membership, the new applicant is usually required to submit to a face-to-face interview with a senior member. Although the discussion will not focus on the management of a particular case, as in other settings, the interview nevertheless provides an opportunity for assessment of other aspects relevant to physician behavior and performance. The interviewer should have goals clearly in mind. Typically these goals would be to:

- *Identify positive attributes that recommend membership and privileges.* These would include professional skills lacking in the medical staff, a potential or actual patient base that would enhance the census, an understanding of and willingness to participate in the peer review process, and so forth.

- *Provide an opportunity for confidential exchange.* A physician who has had a prior health or disciplinary problem is encouraged by a confidential supportive approach to bring forth the controversial background information. The goal is to develop a collaborative approach where possible, in which such a physician is given an opportunity to make a case for acceptance by the medical staff.
- *Identify gross mental or physical disability inconsistent with requested privileges.* For example, a physician with substantial residual paralysis of an upper extremity would be an unlikely candidate for surgical privileges.
- *Identify a mismatch between privileges requested and training or current practice.* The physician who completed a general internal medicine residency a number of years ago is not likely to qualify for subspecialty privileges such as in cardiology, gastroenterology, and so forth, because recent training and experience requirements have become much more stringent.
- *Reveal service demands or expectations beyond the capacity of the hospital.* Examples include sophisticated tertiary care capability or the expectation or immediate referrals in a crowded specialty.
- *Uncover attitudes or values grossly in conflict with those of the hospital or the medical staff.* For example, some physicians are unable to accept the loss of autonomy implied by the concepts of peer review or managed care.

To achieve these goals, an interview should attempt to elicit specific information in an orderly, though not rigidly structured, way. A well-conducted interview will be in a quiet, informal setting. Although the examiner may have a list of criteria in mind, the check sheet should not be in evidence; nor should the encounter be recorded electronically.

Elements of a structured interview should include:

- A narration of training, experience, special skills, and interests
- A brief personal history
- An explicit statement of the applicant's goal in joining the staff
- An accounting of the applicant's needs and expectations in joining the staff, including equipment, personnel, laboratory and imaging services, and access to referral services or panels
- Physical inspection and mental examination by the interviewer, using his or her professional skills to detect gross mental or physical disability
- Evaluation by interviewer of applicant's communication skills and demeanor under stress or challenge

- General fund of medical and specialty knowledge
- Assessment of attitudes toward peer review, medical staff authority, acceptance of group values, and so forth

The intent of the interview is not to preemptively exclude those with physical impairments or those with different cultural values or ethnic backgrounds. Rather, it is to provide an opportunity to examine the physician under stress and to uncover issues that would make the proposed relationship difficult or impossible. The physician who seeks privileges beyond his or her training or physical capacity is exhibiting judgment problems that are likely to spill over into clinical management. The physician who expresses anger and loses control in contemplation of "efficient quality care" and "accountability" to government or governing bodies constantly may be in hot water with the managed care program of the medical staff. A physician seeking return to practice following absence for drug rehabilitation or recovery from serious illness will warrant special evaluation and monitoring as part of a specially tailored, structured reentry plan.

On completion of the interview, the examiner must record the findings in an accepted format, as shown in figure 3-1, and, with his or her evaluation and recommendation, forward them to the appropriate medical staff review body. This report should be made promptly, objectively, and consistently, to minimize the possibility of observer bias.

Provisional Monitoring or Proctoring

When a physician is granted privileges by a medical staff, at best the latter is making an educated guess. The historical information obtained in the credentialing process allows the clinical department or executive committee to make assumptions about a physician's skill based on training, experience, and privileges in other settings. The information is refined by the effort to collect counterbalancing (negative) data from insurance carriers and licensing agencies. The aggregate is analyzed, but at best the yield is a gross correlation between recorded experience and privileges requested. Even a detailed roster of cases successfully performed during a training program gives only a positive prognosis rather than assurance of performance in the hospital setting. By the same token, a prior history of malpractice or chemical dependency is not necessarily a basis for automatic exclusion.

Because of these limitations in the credentialing process, medical staffs have adopted a provisional approach to privilege assignment where physicians are directly observed during their initial exercise of privileges. This process of proctoring, monitoring, or observation may be time-specific, say six months, or procedure-specific, as in five major and five

Figure 3-1. Interview Format

Name of applicant _____

Date of interview _____

Goals in joining medical staff _____

_____

_____

Special practice needs

  Equipment _____

  Personnel _____

  Facilities _____

Special health problems _____

Evaluation of applicant by interviewer

  Physical health—note gross abnormality _____

  Mental health—note gross abnormality _____

  Expressed attitudes toward

    Peer review _____

    Authority of medical staff _____

    Utilization management _____

  General fund of knowledge

    Appropriate to specialty (yes or no) _____

    If no, document observed lack _____

_____

Grade on a scale of 1 to 10 with 10 being most suitable and 1 least suitable for membership _____

_____

_____

minor clinical problems unique to the specialty. Either is appropriate so long as the observed procedures are sufficiently complex to show the skills of the practitioner. At least in some states, accrediting agencies have come to expect that all categories of physicians will be proctored and that a physician's credential file will include reports of the cases reviewed. Departmental and Medical Executive Committee minutes must reflect the successful completion of proctoring. Where a proctored case has been performed poorly, the medical staff is expected to modify or deny requested privileges and/or impose additional training requirements.

Medical Staff Proctoring Policy

Proctoring should be based on an explicit medical staff policy that addresses the following principles:

- The number and complexity of cases should be sufficient to show the physician to be competent in a representative sample of the privileges requested. It is not necessary to proctor every procedure. The proctoring requirement should not be so burdensome as to constitute a means of screening out competition.
- Proctoring should be concurrent where possible. If not, it should be retrospective while the case is still current.
- Proctoring should include the complete management of the patient, not just the procedure.
- The proctor should be a passive observer of care, not a consultant or assistant. There should be no economic relationship between the applicant and the proctor.
- The proctor should have no relationship to the patient. There is no duty for care other than that imposed by the medical staff, which can require the proctor to intervene if the applicant physician is grossly negligent, incompetent, or dangerous.
- The proctor is obligated to report objectively in writing on a prescribed form, within a mandated time. If the care is grossly mishandled or if the proctor had to intervene, the case must be reported immediately to the medical staff authority for consideration of summary revocation of privileges.
- There should be no conflict of interest. The proctor may be a competitor, but there should be no history of overt conflict. There should be several proctors before the applicant completes the requirement. The proctor should not be compensated if he or she is a member of the medical staff.
- If the proctor and the applicant enjoy equivalent privileges at another hospital, some care can be credited if the work is done at the second hospital. Some cases must be performed and proctored at the hospital applied to because physicians may act differently in different facilities.
- The proctor is covered as an observer by the medical staff coverage for peer review. If the proctor intervenes as a consultant or assistant, personal professional liability insurance must be provided. If the proctor intervenes as a good samaritan, individual states may allow for liability exemption, but in most instances coverage again is a matter of personal responsibility.
- There should be no exceptions; everyone should be proctored. At times an unaffiliated proctor in the same specialty is unavailable. In that case, allowing partial credit toward completion may be granted for a proctoring report completed by an assistant, a consultant, or a physician in a different or loosely related specialty. Even the observations of the operating room nurses or anesthesiologist may be better than none at all.

The temptation to make an exception of a professionally or politically powerful physician should be resisted. It is not worth the disruption of an evenhanded proctoring policy. Occasionally, the physician may not live up to advance billing.

Departmental proctoring requirements commonly found in hospitals with well-developed programs encompass all specialties (see figure 3-2). Even radiologists and pathologists are included. For all physicians an effort is made to assess cognitive as well as procedural skills. Figure 3-3 shows a typical reporting form for use by an observer monitoring invasive procedures. The observer is expected to evaluate the indications for the procedure, including assessment of alternatives. Performance is directly viewed, but the proctoring is not complete without consideration of outcome, including recognition and management of complications.

Proctoring a specific procedure is deceptively easy and in many programs constitutes the total review. Concurrent proctoring of cognitive activities without direct intrusion is more difficult. Usually one finds that the work of non-procedure–performing physicians is looked at by a combination of concurrent review of images and laboratory procedures and retrospective review of the record. In the nontraining setting, reexamination of the patient by the proctor is rare. Figures 3-4 and 3-5 list the elements usually included in proctoring programs for primary care and for psychiatry or chemical dependency, respectively.

Proctoring is not without its problems. There is always a tension between the proctor and the proctored. Medical staffs have sought to ease the process by establishing policies that recognize the interests of each party. Executive committees must guard against obvious conflict of interest or anticompetitive activity.

For the peer review process, the information obtained is of unique value and may be clearly determinative. A physician who performs a procedure or manages a case with quiet, efficient competence can be readily recognized. It takes few repeat performances to be able to predict a pattern that would allow continued exercise of privileges without further direct observation. At the other extreme, a physician who commits a clinical error that he or she does not recognize or for which the corrective response is equally inappropriate is immediately perceived as a poor risk. Note in figure 3-3 the requirement to report all failed or poorly executed cases to the medical director (or department chairman). If the error is severe enough, the physician may not get another chance. Similarly, a physician observed to be drunk or "spaced out" on drugs while proctored is likely to be rejected for permanent privileges. Fortunately, most physicians perform well enough to be recognized as a safe risk for assignment of permanent privileges, and the proctoring requirement is terminated.

Figure 3-2. Observation Program

1. Each new medical staff member shall be observed for a minimum of the following:

Family Practice Department
1. First six admissions to the hospital.

Surgery Department
1. First six surgeries including all nonsurgical admissions during Observation Program.

OB/GYN Department
1. First six surgeries including all nonsurgical admissions during Observation Program.
2. First six deliveries.

Pediatric Department
1. First six pediatric admissions to the hospital.
2. First six newborn admissions to the hospital.

Medicine Department
1. First six admissions to the hospital.
2. First six abnormal tracings (EKG).
3. Temporary pacemaker insertion, Swan-Ganz catheter privileges, aortic balloon pumps (three cases, any mix).
4. Treadmill interpretation and monitoring (first six cases).
5. Echocardiogram (first six cases).
6. Upper GI endoscopy (one case), colonoscopy/sigmoidoscopy (one case), polypectomy (one case), laparoscopic liver exam (one case), endoscopic retrograde cholangiopancreatography (one case).
7. Fiberoptic bronchoscopy, percutaneous lung biopsy (first six cases).
8. Renal biopsy (one case).
9. EEG interpretation (first three cases).
10. Peritoneal dialysis (first two cases).
11. Diagnostic and therapeutic cardiac catheterization (five cases).

Anesthesia
1. First six cases.
2. Nurse anesthetists giving obstetrical anesthesia only.
3. First delivery and first four Cesarean sections.

Emergency Room Physician
Emergency medical director evaluates new physicians for a mix of cognitive and procedural skills.

Pathologists and Radiologists
1. Overread of five slides or films.
2. Direct observation of invasive procedures (five cases).

General Rules
1. Reports are submitted within 24 hours of the observation.
2. Observing should be performed by a physician qualified to observe that procedure and who is not involved in a partnership with the physician.
3. The observer should not act as an assistant on surgical cases.
4. The observer should dictate a note or complete an observation sheet/card. The observation notes will become part of the medical staff file.
5. The staff member to be observed is responsible for obtaining a qualified observer. The hospital will provide a list of qualified observers. No one observer should observe more than 40 percent of the required cases.
6. Fifty percent of observed cases can be performed in other hospitals where both the observed and the observer have appropriate privileges.
7. At the completion of the Observation Program, the responsible clinical department will make recommendations as to status of the Observation Program to the Medical Executive Committee.
8. The staff member involved may have his or her name on the referral list in the Emergency Room upon completion of the Observation Program.

Figure 3-3. Procedure Proctoring Report

Please rate categories as follows:

1   Excellent
2   Adequate
3   Marginal
4   Inadequate

Patient name _____

Patient # _____

1. Monitored physician _____
                                          (Name)
2. Monitoring physician _____
                                       (Name or ID #)
3. Procedure _____

4. Date of procedure _____

5. Please answer the following questions: Rating

   Given the clinical picture:

   a. Was the preoperative diagnosis, preparation, and evaluation reasonable?   _____

   b. Was the postoperative diagnosis within a reasonable differential of the preop
      diagnosis?   _____

   c. Was the surgical procedure appropriate to postop diagnosis?   _____

   d. Was the procedure performed adequately technically?   _____

   e. Did intraoperative complications occur?   _____

   f. Were intraoperative complications appropriately handled?   _____

   g. Was the physician's demeanor appropriate?   _____

Please comment on ratings of 3 and 4: _____

_____

Other comments: _____

_____

Overall grade: 1 _____ 2 _____ 3 _____ 4 _____

Dictation of narrative report is optional by the monitoring physician but is suggested, in addition
to completing this form, for all failing ratings.

Notify chief of department or medical director of all failing grades.

Consultation

Outside the training setting, the consultant is the premier peer reviewer.
At the request of the attending physician and the patient, the consultant
is empowered to conduct a thorough independent evaluation of the case.
Usually there is some continuing involvement that permits the consultant an opportunity for longitudinal observation. This intimate involvement allows the consultant an in-depth view of the powers of clinical
observation and integration of the attending physician.

Figure 3-4. Proctoring Elements for Primary Care

1. Admission workup
   - Clear statement of problem
   - Description of outpatient management
   - Supporting data
   - Differential diagnosis
   - Rational working diagnosis

2. Treatment plan
   - Instituted with admission orders
   - Appropriate for working diagnosis
   - Modified according to clinical course
   - Consistent with wishes of patient

3. Treatment process
   - Regular visits documented
   - Appropriate use of consultants
   - Rational drug therapy
   - Monitoring for complications

4. Treatment outcome
   - Discharged to higher or same level of function
   - Satisfactory to patient

5. Special medical procedures

Overall Performance:

_____ Satisfactory _____ Unsatisfactory

Unsatisfactory performance should be immediately reported to the chief of staff.

Why, then, is it rare to find the consultant providing peer review information? By the very intimate nature of involvement the consultant soon ceases to be an objective observer; his or her task is to correct identified clinical deficiencies. If the consultant's judgment process is superimposed on that of the attending physician, the interpretation of events becomes even more complex. If there are five or six consultants, as in the average Medical Intensive Care Unit case, it may be impossible to assign sole responsibility for any event.

Beyond this, consultants are selected for their utility and their compatibility with the practice style of the attending physician. If the latter perceives the consultant as a hostile observer, next time a friendlier adviser will be sought. This is only human nature. The attending physician, unless obligated to choose a specific consultant, will go for the friendly support every time.

Despite these limitations, there are ways of incorporating the observations of consultants into the peer review process:

- *Tabulate reasons for requests for consultation to look for common knowledge or technical deficiencies.* For example, if the consultants in cardiology identify knowledge deficits in the use of new drugs in the management of cardiac arrhythmias among primary care physicians, this information can be reported to the Department of Medicine for incorporation into its continuing medical education program. Group educational programs provide a nonthreatening response to a demonstrated need.

- *Have anesthesiologists log instances of incomplete workup of patients for surgery.* The anesthesiologist also is in a position to identify discrepancies between his or her examination and that of the attending physician or surgeon.
- *Have radiologists track incorrect or redundant sequencing of procedures requested.* By virtue of their review of serial examinations, radiologists are aware of patients who fail to respond or who develop complications following certain procedures.

Figure 3-5. Proctoring Record for Psychiatry or Chemical Dependency

1. Admission workup
   - Clear statement of problem
   - Supporting data
   - Differential diagnosis
   - Working diagnosis—DSM-III

2. Treatment plan
   - Instituted with admission orders
   - Appropriate for working diagnosis
   - Modified according to data

3. Treatment process
   - Regular visits by attending physician documented
   - Appropriate use of consultants
   - Rational drug therapy
   - Patient monitored for effects of drug therapy

4. Treatment outcome
   - Discharged improved
   - Discharged against medical advice
   - Suicide on unit

5. Special psychiatric procedures
   - Electroconvulsive therapy
   - Hypnosis
   - Behavior modification
   - Amytal™ interview

Overall Performance:

_____ Satisfactory _____ Unsatisfactory

Report unsatisfactory grade to evaluating medical director or chief of staff.

- *Have the hospital pharmacist serve as a consultant to physicians regarding drug therapy.* Clinical pharmacy programs achieve a high level of sophistication in recognizing errors in prescribing or dosing medications. By tracking those circumstances in which it is necessary for the pharmacist to intervene because of an error, it is possible to evaluate the prescribing skills of some physicians.
- *Have the emergency staff track unexpected deterioration in patients' conditions.* Many community hospitals maintain an inpatient emergency response service. The physician who responds may be the one who staffs the Emergency Department, or (if the hospital is large enough) there is a dedicated inpatient service. An unexpected deterioration in the patient's condition triggers the emergency consultation if the attending physician is unavailable. A record is maintained of these interventions, usually as part of the cost justification, even if there is no fee-for-service charging by the contract emergency provider. Analysis of that record provides a physician-specific record of unplanned medical catastrophic events. In one hospital such events have included seizures due to unrecognized hypocalcemia, severe hypotension secondary to inadequate fluid replacement in diabetic ketoacidosis, and heart block resulting from digitalis toxicity. Whereas these might be picked up by a generic screening program, to be described in the next chapter, recognition is more precise and immediate by the emergency log analysis. Such information is of value in assessing the skills of both the attending physician and the emergency response physicians.

Emergency service records as just described are not often used, however. The excuse offered is that the attending physician would cease to support the emergency service if it was also part of peer review. This perception is largely political, and an effective medical staff leadership should be able to overcome the objection in the interest of quality of care.

Investigational Monitoring

Not infrequently the medical staff will identify a case that is suggestive of marginal care. Consider a case referred for review because an injury to the spleen occurred during surgery on the descending colon. Analysis by the departmental peer review committee may suggest that the surgeon has a skill or competence deficiency. The single case, however, will be perceived as insufficient to warrant limitation or removal of privileges. Typically, then, the medical staff will impose a requirement that a number of cases be proctored concurrently. Retrospective review of completed cases may also take place, but concern for patient safety and medical staff responsibility adds the concurrent focus. The physician's ability to schedule or admit is not limited, and there is no second opinion requirement. The only imposition is that the physician notify the medical staff office of scheduled surgeries, consultations, and admissions, assuming that the hospital's systems are inadequate to track them on a real-time basis.

Medical staff bylaws usually provide for this option, even though the physician may be long past the initial observational period. The goal of such monitoring is to collect additional data about the overall practice of a physician whose competence is questioned. Information obtained is incorporated as background data in the analysis of a current case or issue. The object of such concurrent investigational proctoring is to make a judgment about the general exercise of privileges in cases not otherwise identified as questionable or to determine whether there is an emerging pattern of poor performance.

Unfortunately, many medical staffs will impose this concurrent proctoring requirement as punitive or corrective action. This defeats the purpose because should there be cause for action, the medical staff would be required to wait for a new case before any action could be taken. Even worse, the proctoring and review requirement becomes a burden for the rest of the medical staff who must do the reviews. In addition, "sentencing" the physician to proctoring as punishment may entitle the physician to formal medical staff appeal rights, and therefore the investigated action could become reportable to state and national discipline data bases.[1]

☐ Limitations of Direct Peer Review

Opportunities for the direct concurrent observation of physician actions are limited. Respect for patient privacy and professional autonomy create barriers that discourage intrusion. The cost of an extra professional solely for surveillance is another limiting factor, even though it may be only the opportunity cost of the lost time that the physician donates. Direct observation also has some of the characteristics of a football game: If you turn your head you may miss the key play; try as you might, you don't always know where the ball is. Direct witnessing of any action is usually recorded only in the mind of the witness. Recall of that record requires some sort of memorization and/or testimony regarding what was seen. Therefore, witnesses are always subject to challenge regarding the accuracy and, hence, the objectivity of their observations. The faithfulness of the record of those observations is also suspect. There is usually no "instant replay" in surgery.

Direct assessment is further limited because it may distort the test situation. Just as in particle physics, where the mere act of observation alters the phenomenon observed, physician and patient behavior may appear different when concurrently monitored. Irascible tyrants may be on their best behavior whereas others, normally callous, may develop white knuckles or sweaty palms. This could be exacerbated should there be a personality clash between the observer and the observed.

Concurrent surveillance (and supervision) is part of the training experience of every physician. Basic maneuvers and complex techniques alike are subject to direct inspection. Cognitive processes are subject to daily or more frequent review by recitation. Clinical actions are second- and third-guessed, all in the interest of training and the accrual of clinical experience at a minimal cost to patient safety. Completion of the training experience leaves this direct intervention and supervision behind. Direct observation, posttraining, brings back the memory and the stress.

Despite these limitations, certain information is best obtained directly. Retrospective analysis of the unwitnessed record (as opposed to the recording of the observations of a witness) will usually miss behavioral traits that may be indicative of an inappropriate reaction to stress. Efficiency and dexterity of hand motion are lost in the dry prose of the procedure report. Concurrent interaction with the physician while he or she is making decisions, judgments, or interpretations may provide a more accurate insight into cognitive skills. A hastily written note in a poor hand by a writer untutored in prose exposition for whom English is a second language may convey little of the clinical data, let alone the intellectual nuance.

☐ Making It Work

Concurrent peer review, then, is feasible, has a distinct role, and is capable of producing information valuable in the assurance of quality. A medical staff that does not take advantage of its opportunities for direct observation of physician practice is grossly deficient in the performance of peer review. This is so despite the acknowledged cost and political, legal, and procedural problems attendant with its use. Procedural problems may be mitigated if the medical staff develops firm policies with at least the following provisions:

- All physicians must undergo direct and concurrent proctoring upon joining the medical staff or upon acquisition of new clinical privileges.
- Conclusion of monitoring on entry does not preclude the reinstitution of direct observation if the physician has had an episode that suggests loss of clinical capacity. Proctoring may be reimposed after a case with an adverse outcome or after prolonged illness or absence of the physician.
- Direct observation per se is not a disciplinary act and does not require either a fair hearing or a report to a state or federal data base.

For reasons of efficiency, medical staffs have been led to develop systems of review that are less immediate, that incorporate screening of large numbers of cases by nonphysicians, and that allow for the more leisurely retrospective analysis of care. Whereas some hospitals rely solely on this method, based on a systematic review of the medical record after discharge, others combine it with concurrent screening while the patient is still hospitalized. The following chapter presents a discussion of criteria-based screening of patient care, retrospective or concurrent—the next essential piece in the peer review mosaic.

□ *Reference*

1. U.S. Department of Health and Human Services, Public Health Service, Health Resources and Services Administration. *National Practitioner Data Bank Guidebook*. Washington, DC: USDHHS, 1990.

Screening Patient Care

There are never enough physicians to review every case, but it is not necessary to have every case reviewed. Professional training and practice standards are strong motivators that, in most instances, ensure an acceptable level of clinical performance. Even without peer review, the average physician will provide good care out of a positive drive to help the patient. Negative constraints and sanctions are tools to control the outlier. Good medical care is not achieved solely by punishments that seek to deter the bad.[1]

Nevertheless, in an era of accountability, it is not sufficient to presume that all care that seems to meet gross clinical standards is acceptable. Using criteria such as the readily recognizable clinical catastrophe (sentinel event), the lawsuit, or the patient complaint, only a few problems will be identified. In the now-famous Medical Insurance Feasibility Study of the California Medical Association and the California Hospital Association,[2] only 1 in 20 of a list of adverse or potentially compensable events was recognized by the patient to the point that a lawsuit was filed. Others have reported similar findings.[3] To rely, then, on the reactions of others to find opportunities for continuous improvement of care is to miss most. Further, it would represent abrogation of responsibility of professionals for self-improvement.

The central element of evaluation of patient care is the review of the patient record. The optimal and definitive method of review remains to be developed; it will evolve as the technology of medical record keeping improves. Paperless systems that provide the same data base for both patient care and its analysis will undoubtedly facilitate review.

140,380

□ Screening of Records by Nonphysicians

The past 20 years have seen the evolution of criteria (the details of which are beyond the scope of this book) for the screening of patient records.

One important development was the publication of generic screening criteria developed by Craddick.[4] These criteria, a sample of which is listed in figure 4-1, represent the centerpiece of most screening systems currently used; they deal with the ultimate outcomes of care or the identification of objective events that might suggest that a clinical process was flawed or that a complication occurred. For example, an unplanned return to surgery or an organ removal may flag either an error in surgical technique or the appropriate management of an unpreventable complication. The goal is to isolate those cases that warrant further review from the total population of patients cared for. The purpose of that review is to identify opportunities for the improvement of patient care or the diminution of factors that threaten patient safety. Flagging the case is not in itself an adverse judgment and without analysis has no peer review judgment value.

In general, review seeks to answer three categories of questions about any procedure or service provided the patient:

1. *Appropriateness.* Given the clinical features of the case, were the right tests and examinations selected? Were the correct conclusions drawn? Were the appropriate treatments applied?
2. *Competence.* Was the care rendered in a professionally competent way? Were interventions timely, well performed, and free of technical error? Were changes in the patient's condition correctly perceived and followed by appropriate modifications in the diagnostic or treatment plan?
3. *Outcome.* Given the severity of the patient's illness at the time treatment began, the acuity of its progression, and the complexity of comorbid conditions, did the patient achieve the optimal outcome that could be reasonably expected?

Screening of care represents the first step in the selection of cases that do not meet standards of appropriateness, competence, or outcome. Figure 4-2 shows examples of screening indicators in each of the three categories.

It is clear from the figure that indicators vary in complexity according to the information sought and the technical nature of the activity being monitored. Typically indicators are applied retrospectively by a trained medical record analyst, after discharge. As a result, the indicators that are likely to be applied will be weighted toward objective events well documented in the medical record. Death, reoperation, and a specialty consultation are readily visible events. Where documentation is incomplete, disorganized, or subjective, the analyst is at a distinct disadvantage. Problems dealing with the quality or efficiency of service, as opposed to outcome, are not easily perceived. Retrospective screening

Figure 4-1. MMA General Outcome Screening Criteria

1. Admission for complications or adverse results of outpatient management

2. Admission for complications or incomplete management of problems on previous hospitalization

3. Operative consent:
   a. Incomplete
   b. Missing prior to procedure
   c. Different procedure
   d. Different surgeon
   e. Not signed
   f. Risks of treatment and alternatives identified during consent process
   g. Other

4. Unplanned removal, injury, or repair of organ or structure during surgery, invasive procedure, or vaginal delivery

5. Unplanned return to operating room on this admission

6. Invasive procedure/tissue:
   a. Pathology report does not match preoperative diagnosis
   b. Nondiagnostic tissue
   c. No tissue removed
   d. Other

7. Transfusion:
   a. Bleeding/anemia, iatrogenic
   b. Not clinically indicated
   c. Transfusion reaction

8. Nosocomial (hospital-acquired) infection

9. Antibiotic/drug utilization

10. Cardiac or respiratory arrest/low Apgar score

11. Transfer from general care to special care unit:
    a. Complication
    b. Utilization problem

12. Other patient complication(s)

13. Hospital-incurred patient incident
    a. Fall
    b. IV problem
    c. Medication error
    d. Skin problem
    e. Other

14. Abnormal laboratory, X-ray, or other test results not addressed by physician

15. Neurological deficit present at discharge that was not present on admission

16. Transfer to another acute care facility

17. Death

18. Subsequent visit to ER or OPD for complication or adverse results related to this hospitalization

Figure 4-2. Examples of Screening Indicators for Appropriateness, Competence, and Outcome

Category of Indicator	Example
Appropriateness	
Blood transfusion	Hemoglobin less than 9 grams
Antibiotics	Organism isolated sensitive to antibiotic
Appendectomy	Inflamed appendix or clinical findings indicative thereof
Competence	
Blood transfusion	No transfusion reaction; pulmonary edema posttransfusion
Antibiotics	Correct dosage; incompatibility avoided; drugs given on time; response to peak and trough drug levels in blood
Appendectomy	Surgery performed before perforation; no intraoperative hemorrhage or organ injury
Outcome	
Blood transfusion	Anemia corrected; cause identified; bleeding stopped
Antibiotics	Culture negative; clinical signs of infection abated
Appendectomy	Length of stay less than 4 days; wound healed primarily; eating normal diet and ambulatory at discharge

also suffers because the analyst typically is not a clinician, although this can be compensated for by a screening policy requiring review by a physician if the data are not clear. A greater deficiency of retrospective review is the inability to apply the observations for the benefit of the patient whose record is being reviewed. Only rarely will postdischarge review be helpful in correcting an error that occurred during the hospitalization.

☐ Concurrent Surveillance

Because of the limitations of retrospective review, many hospitals have added a program that emphasizes concurrent screening of patient care. Utilization review, developed in most hospitals during the Professional Standards Review Organization (PSRO) program for Medicare patients, is a model for a concurrent system.

In a concurrent surveillance system, the goal is to identify potential or actual problems in patient management or outcome in a real-time way. Indicators that screen for appropriateness and efficiency can be tracked in the interest of making service more cost-effective and forestalling inappropriate actions. Where complications occur, concurrent surveillance helps to ensure that the response is timely and correct, so that the ultimate outcome may still be acceptable.

Figure 4-3 illustrates a concurrent surveillance system, where urgent matters receive urgent attention. Less urgent ones may simply be referred for committee review. Each interaction is logged in the quality assurance data base.

Using medical staff indicators a nurse, pharmacist, or technician reviews patient care. In some instances review occurs daily, looking at appropriateness of the clinical regimen and the patient's response. The pharmacist, the nurse, or the technician screens physician orders prospectively. When it is observed that either the order or the patient's status represents a deviation from medical staff standards, the screener confers with a physician adviser who in turn may conduct an independent review. The physician adviser then may either explain the apparent discrepancy or contact the attending physician for more information. In that conversation, the physician adviser may suggest an alternative diagnostic or treatment plan or the need for additional consultation.

In most circumstances, the physician adviser and the attending physician together are able to resolve any differences regarding the patient.

Figure 4-3. Concurrent Surveillance System

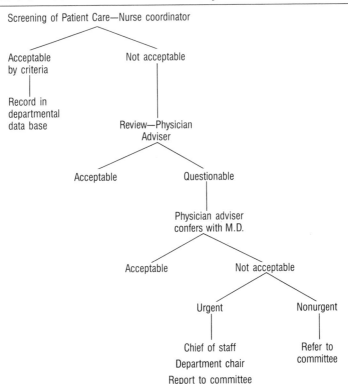

Occasionally, the attending physician will persist in an approach that the physician adviser, after review and discussion, still feels is inherently irrational given the clinical circumstances.

If the situation is urgent, and the contemplated course by the attending physician is likely to result in harm to the patient, the physician adviser is authorized by medical staff policy to contact the chief of staff or respective department chair. The medical staff officer will then intervene with the attending physician. In any event, the nature of the observed discrepancy, the physician adviser evaluation, and the attending physician's response are recorded on a worksheet for review by the Quality Assurance Committee or departmental committee.

Consider the following example. The medical staff has a rule providing that all intensive care unit patients under the care of a primary care physician whose diagnosis is uncertain or in whom there is no therapeutic response within 24 hours must be seen by a specialist consultant, to be chosen by the primary attending physician. This translates into a concurrent indicator "Uncertain diagnosis or failure to improve within 24 hours of admission." The quality assurance nurse coordinator, as part of initial evaluation of appropriateness of ICU admission, notes the criterion and reviews the patient at the end of 24 hours. The nurse may contact the attending physician directly or use a physician quality adviser who would make the call after confirming that the criterion has not been met. The attending physician would be asked to call the appropriate consultant. Refusal by the attending physician to call a consultant could lead to invoking the authority of the department chair or ICU director to enforce the requirement. Unwillingness to comply, especially in the presence of manifest clinical incompetence or impairment, would lead to an ordering of consultation by the director, department chair, or chief of staff.

The first level of screening need not be limited to that performed by a nurse armed with the bedside clinical record. For example, the clinical pharmacist screens drug prescriptions for redundant orders, incompatible combinations, or inadequate or toxic dosages. A record of all drugs ordered and administered is maintained in the pharmacy. Review of the patient's clinical record allows the pharmacist to match the drug order with the patient's clinical findings. If there is a mismatch, the physician is contacted by the pharmacist. After discussion, or clarification in the patient's chart, if the pharmacist's concerns about inappropriate or hazardous drug use are not satisfied, the chairman of the Pharmacy and Therapeutics Committee may be asked to contact the attending physician either to elicit more information or to emphasize the need for a change in the orders.

To illustrate, consider a patient with a chronic urinary tract infection and renal failure. The attending physician orders an aminoglycoside agent that has a potential to aggravate the renal failure, in a dosage that does not account for the decreased ability of the patient to eliminate the drug. Upon contacting the attending physician, the pharmacist is told, "That's the dose I always use. Give the drug. You have no right to question my order." Instead of continuing the debate, the pharmacist would ask the appropriate committee chair or medical staff officer to contact the physician to get an explanation, doctor to doctor, for the unusual drug order. Usually, the discussion leads to appropriate adjustment of the dosage, but the authority of the medical staff to order the pharmacist not to fill the prescription, to substitute another dose or drug, to mandate a consultation by another physician, or even to suspend the physician from the case is implicit in the exchange.

Consider another example. A patient is admitted to an ICU with bleeding from the gastrointestinal tract. After administration of four units of packed red blood cells, the blood pressure remains borderline low; the patient is mildly confused and has a low urine output. The primary care physician in attendance orders additional blood transfusions. Concurrent review of the patient's record by the quality assurance nurse coordinator shows:

- Failure to order blood clotting studies to rule out a bleeding disorder
- Failure to order consultation by an endoscopist or general surgeon to institute definitive care to stop the bleeding
- An order for an upper GI series with barium

The coordinator is authorized by medical staff policy to contact the attending physician. Without further intervention, the appropriate lab tests and consultants are ordered and the X-ray examination is deferred until a more rational management program is agreed on. Although the exchange was between nurse reviewer and attending physician, the action was concurrent peer review as authorized by the medical staff. Most medical staffs will allow for the direct contact between nurse and physician, if only informally. Many review plans retain the requirement that another physician must call the attending physician in this circumstance. The result may be delay, but some attending physicians are still reluctant to accept questions—let alone criticism or restraint—from a nonphysician. Direct communication from the nurse to the attending physician becomes easier with time and credible practice.

Several other illustrations of concurrent screening in the hospital should be noted. Rehabilitation services, particularly those seeking reimbursement for the care of Medicare patients, were offered the opportunity to provide services under precise utilization and appropriateness guidelines in exchange for exemption from prospective payment using diagnosis-related groups (DRGs). The lure of continued cost-plus reimbursement was sufficiently strong to permit medical staffs to adopt strict pretreatment screening criteria applied by rehabilitation specialists to exclude from care the referrals from other physicians that would not qualify for payment. Patients who cannot benefit from intensive rehabilitation because of debility or complicating medical disease are spared the stress and risk. Patients whose neurologic or orthopedic disorder is so advanced as to be chronic and stable at a low level of function are not exposed to the trauma of a vain effort. Those whose impairment is minimal are encouraged to find care in a less expensive outpatient setting. Adherence to these utilization screens ensures continued exempt status. Failure to do so risks significant financial penalties.

Medical staffs have recognized that some diagnostic procedures are sufficiently specialized that the indications for their performance must be controlled. Consider a patient with significant signs of inadequate blood flow to the brain. A vascular surgical procedure, such as a carotid endarterectomy, might be contemplated by the primary care attending physician. An order for X-ray visualization of the cerebral circulation is generated. The radiologist receiving such an order is appropriately concerned about the risk of the procedure. To justify the procedure, the indications clearly must be part of a well-thought-out treatment plan. Because the surgery is beyond the privileges of the primary care physician and the determination of the indications for it may exceed the physician's diagnostic skills, before accepting such an order, the radiologist in some hospitals would want a confirmation of the order by a consulting neurologist or vascular surgeon. Absent such confirmation, the test would not be performed.

Screening of orders for imaging where there are a variety of options is another illustration. For example, a problem in the right upper quadrant of the abdomen might be addressed by:

- Plain film radiography
- Ultrasound
- Isotope biliary excretion studies
- Iodinated contrast studies of the biliary tree and gallbladder
- Isotope scanning of the liver
- Barium contrast studies of the upper and lower intestinal tract
- Iodinated contrast studies of the kidney and urinary tract
- Computerized tomography with and without contrast
- Magnetic resonance imaging

This list is not exclusive. Without going into further clinical detail, it makes the point that one can approach a clinical problem with modalities that may be redundant or dangerous. If ordered in an improper sequence, such as starting with the barium studies, further workup may be precluded until the contrast medium is eliminated. The clinical status of the patient, including acuity and severity, would also influence the choice. A well-run radiology department will review the order in the context of the clinical circumstances and might alter the sequence as part of its peer consultation responsibility.

☐ Automated Systems of Screening

Protection of the patient is a valuable and achievable goal of concurrent screening systems. However, as seen from the preceding examples, nurse and pharmacist review and physician intervention are costly and labor-intensive. Relative to the total number screened, the cases of only a few patients are so identified. A record of such cases would contain only a limited number of entries and, though potentially important, it would be an inadequate and often inaccurate picture of the total practice of a physician. To be more precise, it would be necessary to know the total number of cases a physician cares for, the mix of clinical conditions, the severity of each patient as indicated by the stage of the disease, and the presence of complicating or comorbid illnesses. Comparison with peers on the medical staff would be possible only if this information existed for every physician in the hospital. Comparison among hospitals could occur only if aggregate performance data were collected in each and then shared.

A number of automated systems have been designed to achieve these ends. It must be borne in mind that none of these automated systems is a substitute for an assertive program of concurrent screening and intervention. Instead they are supplemental, for the purpose of collecting aggregate experience retrospectively, looking for patterns of substandard care. Occasionally these systems will identify a severe or "sentinel" case that escaped the concurrent system; that case would be flagged for individual review. More commonly, cases might be found retrospectively that fail to meet less dramatic clinical care criteria; these cases would also be referred for physician review. This individual review or exception analysis will be detailed further in the next chapter.

General Computerized Systems

A computerized system of tracking, screening, and review activity is an essential support for an effective peer review process. Quality assurance and risk management systems depend on data processing and will therefore vary according to the software program that controls them. In general, these systems will seek to provide many or all of the following functions:

- Infection surveillance
- Drug usage evaluation
- Blood usage evaluation
- Surgical case review
- Monitoring and evaluation
- Indicators
- Thresholds
- Physician demographics
- Privileging and credentials
- Identification of cases for review
- Results of the peer review process
- Incident/occurrence monitoring
- Severity-of-illness indexing
- Utilization review
- Risk management
- DRG and other coding

This list was adapted from the questionnaire for vendors in *How to Buy QA/RM Software* by Shanahan and Hopkins.[5] Readers interested in evaluating or acquiring a computerized system should consult that work for a detailed list of available (as of 1988) systems. Because the many available systems are undergoing constant review and modification, individual vendors should be consulted. Most will provide substantial assistance to the medical staff seeking to make its peer review processes more automated and more comprehensive.

Risk Adjustment Systems

As yet, there is no ideal system for comparing patients according to the severity of their primary disease or the effect of preexisting comorbidities or treatment complications. Systems that log objective data from clinical, laboratory, and X-ray examinations can provide a basis for the comparison of groups of patients. In the aggregate, these and similar data can characterize a patient population within a hospital or a group of hospitals. As such they are epidemiologic tools. With further refinement, they will be useful to evaluate the effectiveness of various medical management approaches on the outcome of care, as well as the reliability and consistency of individual hospitals or systems. Where one physician in a hospital is responsible for all examples of a particular type of case or procedure, the data could reflect that physician's performance as well.

Six systems are currently marketed. For a detailed comparison see the work by Geehr[6] on selecting a proprietary severity-of-illness system. Other evaluations of the role of risk adjustment systems confirm that peer review of the individual case is likely to remain the ultimate means of the judgment of quality for some time to come.[7]

Performance Profiles Data Base

Some hospitals have succeeded in developing physician profiles that log the use of individual ancillary services, such as X rays and laboratory tests, by disease category or DRG.[8,9] Consider two physicians, each of whom has performed 10 appendectomies for acute appendicitis without rupture. Physician use pattern shows the following per case:

	Dr. A	Dr. B
Complete blood counts	2.0	4.0
ICU days	0.1	1.2
Abdominal X rays	.4	2.0
Wound cultures	.1	4.0

These da\. either reflect different practice patterns or a different case mix due to adv_ e selection or poor performance. Presentation of the data to the physician encourages evaluation of the depicted practice pattern. From that self-assessment can come the motivation for practice modification.

As the DRG system becomes refined by adding factors of severity, stage, and comorbidity, profiling of the physician by resource use will become even more valuable. Availability of reliable profiles has permitted physicians in some hospitals to compare their performance with their peers in the interest of self-correction. For the moment, and in the foreseeable future, data-based performance profiles will be dependent on the analysis of exceptional records by physicians trained to look for the clinical nuances, which as yet are not captured by automated systems.[10,11]

Chapter 5 presents a system for review of individual records identified as exceptional by medical screening procedures. In chapter 6 the use of this information, along with other aggregate data to create comparisons and detect trends of physician performance, will be described.

☐ *References*

1. Berwick, D. M. Continuous improvement as an ideal in health care. *New England Journal of Medicine* 320(1):53–56, Jan. 5, 1989.
2. *CMA/CHA Medical Insurance Feasibility Study.* San Francisco: Sutter Publications, 1977.

3. Brennan, T. A., and others. Identification of adverse events during hospitalization. *Annals of Internal Medicine* 112(3):221-26, Feb. 1, 1990.

4. Craddick, J. W. *Medical Management Analysis: A Systematic Approach to Quality Assurance.* Auburn, CA: J. W. Craddick, 1983.

5. Shanahan, M. A., and Hopkins, J. L. *How to Buy QA/RM Software.* Chicago: Joint Commission on Accreditation of Healthcare Organizations, 1988.

6. Geehr, E. C. Selecting a proprietary severity of illness system. American College of Physician Executives, Tampa, 1989.

7. Goldschmidt, P. G. Red herring or horse of a different color? Part I. *Physician Executive* 15(4), July–Aug. 1989.

8. Schapiro, A. DRG reimbursement and physician management. *QRC Advisor* 6(1):3-8, Nov. 1989.

9. Eisenberg, J. M. Doctors' decisions and the cost of medical care. *Health Administration Press Perspectives.* Ann Arbor, MI: Health Administration Press, 1986.

10. Goldfield, N., and Nach, D. B., editors. *Providing Quality Care.* Philadelphia: American College of Physicians, 1989.

11. Economic credentialing is fine—for tightrope walkers. *Hospital Peer Review* 15(4):49-68, Apr. 1990.

Exception Analysis by Physicians

The traditional approach to peer review identifies the individual case for focused physician analysis. This exceptional event would be detected by the screening of care described in chapter 4. In setting up such a system, the medical staff would identify which cases mandated individual chart review. Records so designated are analyzed by physicians with equivalent professional skill (see chapter 2, "Definition of a Peer"). The analysis seeks to expose the intellectual processes that led to the clinical decision making evidenced by the record. The object is to identify opportunities for self-improvement and, secondarily, to identify those physicians who might need help in future cases. From time to time (not often enough in the minds of some) an event reflecting gross negligence or incompetence would be uncovered.[1-3] Limiting the clinical privileges of the physician responsible might follow. Clearly, then, a chart identified for peer review might be a serious career-limiting event.

Physicians, at the core, have strong egos. Professional success requires the ability to take dangerous action in the face of incomplete data and be right most of the time.[4] If the action proves wrong, the range of error must be narrow, reflecting reasonable clinical choice where the preponderance of information did not indicate a particular direction. The right to clinical decision making under such circumstances is a key ingredient of physician autonomy. The autonomous physician sincerely feels he or she has no peers in a given clinical situation and, therefore, that peer review is inherently deficient as a process. Arguments in support of this position run something like this:

- My experience is unique, my training special. Only I can understand all of the clinical facts in the case.
- I have been following this patient for 20 years. I know what he or she was really saying.

- Regardless of clinical indications, I know the family. They never would have consented to the procedure.
- Because so few of us specialize in such cases, any review of my work will be biased. Physicians reviewing my cases benefit economically from "exposing my failures."

Thus, peer review is always perceived as a threat to the ego and the autonomous rights and privileges of the physician. Effective peer review requires the recognition of this challenge. Motivation of effective peer review, to be discussed in greater depth in chapter 9, is one answer to such challenges. This chapter focuses on the process of peer review as one approach to blunting the challenge.

☐ Achieving Fair Peer Review

Inherent in criticism of peer review is its imputed unfairness. Physicians are quick to assert that a case was pulled capriciously whereas similar cases escaped detection or were deliberately overlooked. Bias in chart selection is clearly a possibility, the result of malice or economic or personal gain. It may also be the result of prior review. That is, a physician identified as having had a problem case will have earned "name recognition" so that every case thereafter may be suspect on its face.

Case selection for peer analysis, therefore, must stand the challenge of fairness. Initial attempts sought to achieve fairness by a process of random selection. Designation of every 10th or 20th case using a random number table was a common approach that may still be used in some settings. It satisfies the test of objectivity of selection but fails in two important areas. By its randomness it will select a number of cases that have no problems and from which little if anything is gained by the review. Similarly, the random approach will miss many problems, allowing the unfairness argument to assert "my case was reviewed while others were ignored."

For these reasons random screening, though fair in its application, is unfair in its results. Greater fairness can be achieved by identifying the objective criteria that characterize all cases that merit review, solely because those criteria are met.[5] To illustrate, then, a screening system will usually provide that all cases in which patients die are subjected to such review. Death is an adverse event signaling failure of therapeutic interventions and therefore is worthy of serious analysis. Unfortunately, this view leads to the review of many cases in which death was inevitable. Because in every hospital death is a common event, many records are flagged and much time is expended, often for little yield. As a consequence, some medical staffs focus their attention on cases in which death was unexpected, such as after elective surgery or nonlethal illness. Other examples of cases that could be excluded in the screening process from the general category of death are:

- Patients over age 90 with advanced terminal neurologic disease, four extremity contractures, and decubitus ulcers
- Patients previously hospitalized and reviewed with known terminal disease beyond the scope of treatment
- Patients who suffer cardiopulmonary arrest "in the field" who are resuscitated in the emergency room to the level of ventilator dependency and serious anoxic brain damage

Each of these categories might be a subject for focused study at prescribed intervals. However, their elimination from the general exception analysis of mortality cases would free scarce physician reviewer time for more potentially significant cases.

Modern occurrence screens will flag cases for review for a variety of reasons, limited only by the resources and interests of the medical staff. Indicators of charts for exception analysis may be related to risk in general—such as all patients admitted to a critical care unit after a surgical procedure not usually requiring that level of care. In that example, the screen would flag a case in which an unexpected complication or degree of severity of illness was encountered. Indicators may also be specific and precise, such as all patients treated with parenteral antihypertensive drugs for accelerated or severe hypertension whose blood pressure after 24 hours is above 200/120 or below 110/60. The goal of this indicator would be to select for exception analysis those cases of severe high blood pressure that were potentially overtreated or undertreated during a critical phase of the patient's illness.

One can see from these two examples that indicators vary in specificity. Either extreme is appropriate, given the proper circumstance, so long as the event that flags the case for review is measurable as part of the regular processes of patient care. Because admission to a critical care unit and measurement of blood pressure are basic nursing care functions, their notation requires no special intervention. All cases would be identified as part of standard patient care practice. Thereby, the system of exceptional chart identification would be both fair and objective.

In the concurrent screening system depicted in chapter 4, figure 4-3, a nonphysician uses medical staff screening criteria to flag cases for physician review. This process is equally applicable to retrospective review. Screening in this circumstance is performed by medical record or quality assurance personnel. Whether the case is a nonurgent one coming from the concurrent system or a retrospective one, most medical staffs find it prudent to subject the record that is flagged to a physician screening review. The goal of the physician screener is to acquire the essential facts in summary detail and, based on them, decide whether to refer the case for possible medical staff action. Physician screeners are often reluctant to participate in this process. However, if the responsibility is shared and their activities, by policy and action, are supported by the medical staff organization, department members will usually come forward. With appropriate support and training, screening can achieve the twin goals of consistency and efficiency necessary for effective conduct.

☐ Focused Peer Review

Several tools are available to the medical staff to achieve consistency and efficiency in physician screening activities. The first is standardization of the review process, attained by obliging the screener to answer a specific set of questions about each case. The second is the development of criteria for referring a case for definitive action.

Standardization of the Review Process

The following questions, which appear on the peer review worksheet shown in figure 5-1, point the reviewer to the specific concerns raised by the event that caused the case to fall out of the screening process:

1. *What was the identified clinical event?* The referral from the nurse or record room screener will identify the indicator or criterion that led to the chart referral. The physician reviewer, after completion of chart analysis, is asked to recast the reason for referral in more precise clinical terms. Thus a referral for "patient fall with injury" might be described by the physician as "postural hypotension leading to syncope, resulting in a fall causing an intertrochanteric fracture of the left hip."
2. *Was the care rendered prior to the event responsible for its occurrence?* The physician is asked to identify the causes for the event and their relationship to it. For the patient injury described under question #1, the answer might be that despite orders for antihypertensive drugs, vasodilators for cold feet, sleeping pills, and tranquilizers, there was no order to measure the patient's blood pressure in the erect position or for nursing to assist the patient while ambulating.
3. *Was care below the community standard?* The question seeks to commit the screening physician to an evaluation of the events that led to the incident. In practice, this question has led to expressions of physician resistance to attributing any meaning to a nebulous community standard. Furthermore, it is perceived among physicians as highly judgmental and therefore carries substantial political and legal liability. Note

Figure 5-1. Peer Review Form: Confidential Medical Staff Information

Section I

Patient _____   Medical record # _____

Date of admission _____   Admitting MD # _____

Reason for referral: (State specific indicator, criterion, or other reason for review.) _____

Section II (Please answer all questions.)

1. What was the identified clinical event? _____

2. Was the care rendered prior to the event responsible for its occurrence? _____

3. Did the care deviate sufficiently from standards of care to warrant further review?

   _____ Yes _____ No

4. Was a specific practitioner responsible for the event requiring review?

   _____ Yes _____ No   Medical staff # _____

5. What specific actions were performed or omitted that contributed to the event or the patient's disposition? _____

6. Would a practitioner with similar clinical privileges be expected to avoid or manage the clinical event differently? _____

7. Was death or major disability a result of this event? _____ Yes _____ No

Section III

1. Was the documentation in the chart clinically pertinent to the patient's condition and treatment?

   _____ Yes _____ No

   If no, cite specific references _____

2. Was the chart documentation sufficient for your review? _____ Yes _____ No

   If no, which items were missing:

   _____ History and physical   _____ Discharge summary

   _____ Operative report   _____ Consultant reports

   _____ Progress notes (Cite dates missing)_____

   Comments _____

   _____   _____
   Reviewer's signature   Date of review

Section IV

Decision of Department Committee or Review Committee

_____ Is there a pattern of similar events?   _____ Refer for documentation

_____ Referral to department for further review   _____ Letter of inquiry

_____ Approval with no action

_____   _____
Reviewing committee   Date of review

that this question has been rephrased in question 3 of the peer review worksheet (figure 5-1) as, "Did the care deviate sufficiently from standards of care to warrant further review?" This is substantially the same question, but it relieves the screening physician of the burden of first judgment of failure to meet community standards.

4. *Was a specific practitioner responsible for the event requiring review?* In our example, one can attribute responsibility to a single physician for drug and blood pressure orders. The value of this in peer review is self-evident. The question becomes much more complex with regard to a patient in a critical care unit where six different medical subspecialists write orders that might influence patient blood pressure. In that instance, the screening physician might identify the failure to designate a single physician case manager as the causal omission.

5. *What specific actions were performed or omitted?* This question seeks to obtain a precise clinical statement from the screening physician. Initially it may be perceived as redundant, but its answer focuses the clinical department discussion on specialty-specific performance. It also serves as the basis for a specific statement of charges, should some restrictive action eventuate. In our example, failure to order blood pressure measurements in the erect position would be one critical act of omission. Prescribing too many drugs might be another action.

6. *Would a practitioner with similar clinical privileges be expected to avoid the event?* This question is another approach to the issue of practice standards. It does not seek a precise measure but rather an opinion from a peer. Where the causal action or omission is highly specialized, such as failure to employ a specific surgical or complex medical approach, the answer might indicate that the screener lacks the skill to make a valid judgment. In that case, a second specialty review would be indicated prior to or as part of departmental review. On the other hand, where the omission involves more basic and universal medical knowledge, highly specialized peer review is not an essential at this level. Any physician should know that certain commonly used drugs interfere with blood pressure regulation and, therefore, that monitoring is indicated.

7. *Was death or major disability a result of this event?* This information flags cases that on the face warrant more intensive review because of their high visibility and high risk to institutional reputation and resources.

8. *Is there a pattern of similar clinical events associated with care below standard?* The screening physician may not know the answer here. The question is included (in section IV) to direct the reviewing department to explore that issue before concluding its analysis.

Upon completion of the form in figure 5-1, screening physicians may still be reluctant to refer the case for definitive departmental review. In the mind of the physician whose case it is, such referral is tantamount to an adverse judgment. Litigious physicians have sought to involve their personal attorneys at this point in an effort to block referral. Tactics may include reference to the bylaws, but more commonly intimidation is invoked. The screener refers a case under implied threat of lawsuit. Less severely, the reviewer may simply risk friendship or a referral source.

Criteria for Referral for Definitive Action

The medical staff can come to the aid of the screening physician by adopting criteria that mandate referral from the first-level physician screening to the definitive review and action levels. Use of these criteria allows the screener the defense of being merely a finder of fact. If certain facts are present, then referral is mandated by medical staff policy. No one would expect the screener to hide or purposely overlook certain facts. Thus, the action of referral represents an automatic expression of medical staff policy and not a personal act of individual clinical judgment.

Criteria that mandate referral from the screening to the definitive review level might include the following elements:

- Event associated with death
- Event associated with major injury
- Event associated with a specific problem in physician technique or judgment
- Event associated with a physician exceeding his or her clinical privileges
- Event associated with a patient complaint, lawsuit, or citation
- One of a series of problems known to be associated with the same physician
- One of a series of similar events involving different physicians
- Event associated with complications requiring significantly increased care

The use of screening criteria for referral achieves several valuable ends:

- It ensures that serious cases come to the attention of the definitive review body.
- It avoids wasting valuable committee time spent screening randomly or looking at minor events.
- It emphasizes peer review as a serious business dealing with problems that threaten patient safety and professional integrity.

☐ Evaluating and Training Peer Reviewers

Departments are obliged to assess the quality of work done by peer reviewers. A regular program of evaluation emphasizes the meaning and value of the process. Analysis of the errors observed allows for focused training of reviewers. Physicians incapable of performing objective, efficient review may be precluded from participation. Physicians qualified for review may be singled out for special recognition.

Evaluating Peer Reviewers

A departmental assessment of the performance of its peer reviewers might find the following kinds of problems:

- *Delayed review.* Often seen in retrospective systems where there seems to be no urgency to screen or review. The result may be lack of enthusiasm because the cases are old and dry.
- *Superficial review.* Physicians usually review in their spare time. As the physician's practice (earning a living) comes first, he or she may only skim the record.
- *Underevaluation.* In part this is a sign of superficial review. It may also result from an unwillingness of the reviewer to get involved by addressing hard questions.
- *Overevaluation.* An unusual amount of detail or an unwillingness to accept obvious exculpatory evidence may indicate a personal bias on the part of the reviewer or a hostile motivation for the review.
- *Unfocused responsibility.* Although this may just reflect superficial analysis, it may indicate that the reviewer is unwilling to "finger" a colleague.
- *Projected responsibility.* A common response to a case suggestive of physician failure is to identify potential hospital factors that may be at fault. Thus, for the patient with the hip fracture described earlier, emphasis might be placed on the failure of nursing policy to mandate erect blood pressure checks or assisted ambulation rather than the assignment of specific responsibility to the physician for failure to write the precautionary order. The perverse result of this practice is the expanded role of nursing policy in the direction of patient care. It is, of course, perverse from the point of view of physician autonomy, not necessarily patient safety.
- *Clinically incompetent review.* At times a marginal physician will end up reviewing a superior one in the same specialty. This is a risk especially where primary care physicians review subspecialists who may also do primary work. It may also arise where the cause of the event is due to a breach of specialty technique with which the reviewer is unfamiliar.

- *Undocumented information.* The delinquent medical record, missing key reports such as a history and physical, operation, or consultation, may be unreviewable until the missing data are supplied (see figure 5-1). On the other hand, in the focused chart review of the patient who fell (described earlier), absence of a consult from the rehabilitation service, postfracture, has no bearing on the analysis of the cause of the fall. That absence may be a separate cause for medical staff action (or improvement of medical records processing by the hospital). Completion of the hip fracture analysis, for example, should not be delayed by the jurisdictional dispute.
- *Charitable second-guesses.* Physician reviewers are tempted to supply the data missing from a record, by inference. For example, if the basis for a physician's decision is not clear, it is likely the benefit of the doubt will be given, based on "We know Joe! He wouldn't make that mistake." A better principle is the one developed in the early days of utilization review: If it wasn't documented it didn't happen, unless it can be proven from other records from the physician's office. Here reviewer creativity may be required; it may be acceptable to conclude that a physician included diabetes in his differential diagnosis based on the blood sugar done in the preadmission chemistry panel.

Training Peer Reviewers

Training physicians to perform exception analysis should include a review of the common clinical performance errors that might be uncovered. Examples of such errors might include:

- Failure to respond to abnormal clinical or laboratory data
- Commission or omission in making a diagnostic error
- Selecting the wrong treatment modality or regimen
- Incompetent performance of a treatment or procedure
- Failure to monitor the appropriate diagnostic or treatment parameters
- Failure to respond to clinical circumstances with appropriate diagnostic or treatment intensity; premature termination of treatment or prolongation of treatment to the point of harm
- Uncontrolled events that led to adverse outcome because of comorbidity
- Clinical circumstances requiring intervention beyond the state of the art in a particular setting

Specific details of these issues in a given situation will depend on the clinical skill and judgment of the reviewer. Often these clinical points will be the focus for discussion at subsequent levels of review. The reviewer should be encouraged to be specific and detailed in the initial screening.

The physician reviewer should also be alerted to the differences in findings of the clinician during life and the pathologist at autopsy. Autopsies continue to reveal missed diagnoses despite modern imaging and biochemical techniques. The task of the clinical reviewer is to judge whether the attending physician should have made the diagnosis antemortem. Autopsies have declined in number and importance as a result of reimbursement changes. Nonetheless, the Joint Commission on Accreditation of Healthcare Organizations (JCAHO) emphasizes that the medical staff must include the results of autopsies in its peer review process. Where there is diagnostic uncertainty, therapeutic question, or where death was not anticipated, autopsies should be sought to help the objectivity and intensity of peer review.[6] Issues identified in the preceding list may have a fatal expression.

☐ Definitive Review and Action

If the screening process identifies a problem in which further review is mandated, the record and the recorded observations of the physician are submitted for definitive review and action. Review may take place in an open departmental meeting (or a meeting of the staff as a whole if the hospital is small) if the case is straightforward, of educational value, and is not likely to lead to punitive action. If there are more than a few cases of this type, review is better accomplished by a peer review committee of the staff or department. In that event, a summary report is then presented at the open meeting, including recommendations for action. In general, if a case is "so hot" that restrictive action is seen as likely, confidential discussion of the specific identified event by a peer review or department service committee is preferred. The report to the department, then, may be abstract and anonymous so that the department may escape allegations of defamation or prevention of a fair hearing by biasing department members.

Peer review is not complete without departmental discussion and action. It is not enough to discuss the case in the interest of continuing medical education. Laudable though that activity might be, it is insufficient as peer review conducted in unless the interest of furthering quality care is also served.

Consider the following example. A patient was admitted to the hospital for evaluation of a fever of unknown origin. The patient, who suffers from a blood dyscrasia, underwent extensive outpatient workup for oral temperatures to 102° for two weeks. During the night, after admission, the temperature reached 104°, but by morning rounds it was down to 99.6° and the patient was sent home by the attending physician. Later that day, the patient had to be recalled to the hospital for intravenous antibiotics because two blood cultures were suggestive of a staphylococcus species, indicating sepsis. Despite a satisfactory outcome, the patient's confidence in the doctor and the hospital was seriously shaken in the short run.

The case came for departmental discussion because of the complaint from risk management. Departmental minutes logged three pages of medical debate about the causes of hyperpyrexia in Hodgkin's disease, but no conclusions were reached. None were thought to be required. The purposes of peer review would have been better served if the discussion had focused on five direct questions:

1. What is the clinical circumstance?
2. What was the questioned clinical action?
3. What is the lesson for the individual physician?
4. What is the lesson for the clinical department (or medical staff)?
5. What is the lesson for the hospital?

In our example, the answers are clear:

1. The clinical circumstance was the discharge of a patient prematurely, resulting in inconvenience, risk, and patient dissatisfaction.
2. The questioned clinical action was failure to adequately evaluate a patient before discharge.
3. The lesson for the physician was that one should review the entire temperature record before concluding the fever was down.
4. The lesson for the medical staff was consideration of a standard that says it is inappropriate to discharge a patient who had a temperature of 104° in the previous 24 hours. (Professional Standards Review Organization quality guidelines would call into question a temperature above 101° in that circumstance.)
5. For the hospital, a "panic value" policy for fever above 103°, for example, would have caused the nurse to call the physician, even during the night, for possible additional orders.

Peer review, then, is not complete unless the process, which begins with screening against criteria, concludes with one of three general judgments:

1. The review was not needed because the indicators were met and the referral was in error.
2. The indicators were not met, and some appropriate policy or education is warranted.
3. The indicators were not met, and some restrictive correction action is contemplated.

The appropriate design of corrective action will be detailed in chapter 7.

☐ Departmental Leadership of Peer Review

Implementation of medical staff and quality assurance information systems, coupled with a structured system of exception analysis, signals the end of an era for many hospitals. At some point in the evolution of a hospital, not necessarily in its early stages, a dominant figure may emerge in a particular clinical department. In the author's experience the leader is usually a surgeon, but such leadership is more a function of personality and clinical skill than specialty. The individual quickly becomes the principal departmental consultant. The physician also becomes the resource for administrative problem solving of issues dealing with physicians. In that latter capacity, he or she is called on to intercede if the operating room supervisor anticipated or witnessed a physician performing an inappropriate procedure. This leader is the person called if the administrator is faced with a drunken physician or a lawsuit involving a major loss resulting from surgery. The dominant physician ultimately emerges as a sort of super-peer who is the embodiment of physician regulation, even without the blessings of the medical staff. In some circumstances, the "heroic" physician takes up the "functional space" of the medical staff organization. As a result, the physician might come to dominate the medical staff organization, which regresses into a vestigial appendage. The very effectiveness of the super-peer in controlling the practice in the department, and especially within the surgical suite, is often a deterrent to the development of effective group processes to handle the quality assurance, risk management, peer review, and disciplinary functions that have been usurped.

Heroic super-peers are not to be disparaged. In modern terms, they serve the functions encompassed by the medical director, the department chairman, and the administrative physician responsible for surgery and anesthesia required by the JCAHO. In the concurrent screening system depicted in chapter 4, they would be represented by the physician authority charged with the task of responding to urgent quality problems. Indeed, the current emphasis on the linkage between quality assurance, peer review, and urgent corrective action is an effort to systematize the functions served by this single dominant physician. These group functions may be seen as an outgrowth of those individual efforts.

Despite that, as medical information systems evolve, as quality assurance moves in the direction of ongoing surveillance, and as medical staffs become more sophisticated in the art of objective peer review and privilege allocation, a dysfunctional relationship may emerge between the heroic super-peer and the organized medical staff. The analogy might be Caesar or Hannibal constrained by the Pentagon or the Senate Armed Services Committee. Perforce, growth in the authority of the group processes, whether legislative or bureaucratic, diminishes the autonomy and the authority of the dominant individual physician. The adoption of policies that mandate group instead of personal peer control processes or the identification of other individuals or committees to support administrative problem solving interferes with heroic autonomy. The dominant physician may then pass from the peer review scene. The mode of passage is likely to be a function of his or her clinical and political status at the time. Ideally, the past contributions should be recognized and placed in the historical perspective of the evolution of the medical staff organization. Regrettably, the departure may come late in the career of the super-peer, accompanied by allegations of declining clinical competence.

Departure of the heroic super-peer may leave a gap in the review processes of the medical staff. Particularly, the group must retain ability to respond quickly with authority to forestall a serious clinical failure while the case is salvageable. One of the problems of organization-based authority is that its exercise may require cumbersome and time-consuming deliberation. The medical staff must designate physicians with the stature and authority to perform many of the functions of the super-peer to ensure the operational effectiveness of the clinical department. This differs from the role played by the heroic physician in that the authority for peer evaluation and restraint is not his or her unique personality but the bylaws of the organized medical staff. The ideal mix, of course, would be found in a physician who had the courage and tenacity of the heroic super-peer and the political skills and desire to work within the organized medical staff.

☐ *References*

1. Mills, D. H. Whither malpractice litigation. *Western Journal of Medicine* 149:611–15, 1988.
2. Morlock, L., and others. Malpractice clinical risk management and quality assessment in providing quality care. American College of Physicians, Philadelphia, 1989.
3. *Surgical Case Review: A Quality Assurance Issue.* Chicago: Joint Commission on Accreditation of Healthcare Organizations, 1988.
4. Gerrity, M. S., DeVellis, R. F., and Earp, J. A. Physicians' reactions to uncertainty in patient care. *Medical Care* 28(8):724–36, Aug. 1990.
5. Schultz, R. Making computerized quality assurance work. *QRC Advisor* 6(8):1–8, June 1990.
6. Anderson, R. E. How autopsy can be used in quality assessment. *QA Review* 1(4), Nov. 1989.

Improving Performance through Data Analysis

To date, most medical staffs have taken a minimalist approach to compliance with the requirements for developing physician profiles. Despite the expectations of the JCAHO and Medicare, and the independent efforts of insurance companies to characterize the good provider, medical staffs have only reluctantly gone along. In part, the reluctance has stemmed from the inherent desire to avoid being stereotyped by numbers. More significantly, resistance has come from a concern that practice-limiting decisions will grow out of flawed or imprecise measures.

☐ The Aggregate Performance Profile

Despite their reluctance to develop physician profiles, medical staffs are collecting information regarding physician performance.[1] These data reflect the number of cases that have failed quality assurance screens and, after peer review, have indicated some professional lapse.[2] Typically a physician will have few or none of these in a two-year period. Cases that are identified are likely to be random or unrelated.

The minimally acceptable aggregate performance profile of a physician is likely to contain the following elements:

- Total number of cases as attending physician or surgeon
- Total number of cases as assistant
- Total number of cases as consultant
- Mortality
- Length of stay by diagnostic category
- Total cost by diagnostic category
- Ancillary service cost by diagnostic category

- Number of cases failing quality assurance screen (sorted by indicator)
- Number of cases failing peer review (sorted by indicator)
- Corrective actions taken after peer review
- Total days suspended for medical record violations

These generic data provide some insight into the effectiveness and the efficiency of the practitioner. A profile with these elements would satisfy JCAHO accreditation standards as well as withstand the sometimes harsher scrutiny of a Medicare validation survey. Despite that, medical staffs have not found such profiles to be useful in making credentialing decisions, generally because the elements are not sufficiently focused on performance measures. As the goal of profile analysis is to make an informed projection regarding continued ability to exercise clinical privileges with safety and competence, the clinical department should seek more specific information. A more useful set of elements would add the following to the minimal set:

1. Cases performed as attending physician or surgeon sorted by complexity using standard privileging categories in which, for example, a hernia repair would be level 1, a common bile duct exploration level 3, and so forth.
2. Cases admitted outside a physician's specialty indicating a shift in practice pattern. In combination with data from the first element in this list, these might indicate that a surgeon was scaling down his or her practice for reasons of health or age.
3. Complication rate per specific procedure compared against the department mean and the literature.
4. Resource utilization rate per diagnosis or homogeneous diagnostic category. Rates should be expressed in terms of units of a specific service, such as ICU days, CT scans, or chest X rays, and compared with the departmental mean.
5. Cases denied by outside review agencies.
6. Liability actions.
7. Adverse cases or actions reported to state and federal data banks.

This expanded set of elements would provide even more information about a physician's practice pattern. Tracked over time, one could identify trends that might flag a decline in performance. Sharing the departmental mean gives the physician a basis from which to compare his or her performance with that of peers. Using rates and percentages, one can determine whether a particularly high number of complications is a reflection of skill or merely an indication that the physician is handling a large number of difficult cases. Further refinement in this respect can be achieved by sorting cases according to age or comorbid conditions or by applying one of the propriety severity systems, such as APACHE II, MedisGroups, and so on.

The goal of physician profiling is to determine whether performance is at the department standard. Presumably, the departmental standard is consistent with the broader community standard, as expressed in the specialty literature. Thus a measure of comfort may be derived from the knowledge that the operative mortality rates for a given procedure by the surgeon and the department are the same as those found in good programs elsewhere in the country. From that it is safe to conclude that the physician is practicing at the community standard and that privileges to perform that procedure may be continued during the next two-year reappointment cycle. Aberrant patterns may be shared with the individual physician as they emerge. This is illustrated in the example presented at the end of chapter 4, comparing two surgeons' experience with appendicitis.

□ Productivity Performance Indicators

Peer review based on the community standard identifies the physician who practices at the minimum level of acceptability. Whereas many physicians exceed that level, for some it represents their peak. This is not intended to disparage the physician who practices at the community standard. By definition, that means that, as judged by fellow professionals and the courts, care is appropriate and would likely satisfy patients as well. Even in rural and inner-city settings, most care is at the community standard. Current quality assurance and peer review systems based on generic outcome indicators are inadequate, however, because of their focus on this minimum level of approval. For example, determining that a physician has a rate of postoperative wound infections or gross mortality within 2 standard deviations of his or her peer group provides only the roughest measure of skill or efficiency.

As a result of data that track other performance measures, it is possible to distinguish the better (or best) physician from the adequate (or good) one. This distinction will become more important as medical staffs and physician groups vie for competitive advantage in gaining market share. Consider a straightforward operation, such as an appendectomy for acute appendicitis. Adding additional data that are regularly collected for all appendectomies to that profiled in chapter 4 (physician use per case of CBCs, ICU days, abdominal X rays, wound cultures), one can evaluate how well a physician handles the essential elements in the performance of that procedure. These data could include the following:

- Time from presentation of patient to definitive decision to operate
- Surgical time—skin to skin

- Accuracy rate of diagnosis
- Rate of preoperative or intraoperative perforation
- Length of stay in hospital
- Antibiotics in postoperative period, number of days
- Secondary procedure rate
- Hospital mortality
- Total cost and ancillary service cost of hospitalization

This profile of elements borrows from the work of Steven Lewis, M.D., of Intermountain Health, who has performed similar studies for cholecystectomy and transurethral resection of the prostate.[3] Figure 6-1 provides an adaptation of the indicators used in Lewis's prostatectomy study. That study showed that above the minimum of the community standard, there was a hierarchy of surgeons, all acceptable, but some clearly better than others. In the prostatectomy group, the fastest surgeon had a mean time of 25 minutes; the slowest, 100 minutes. Perhaps not surprisingly, the slower surgeon resected less tissue and had a higher number of patients whose convalescence was marked by a longer duration of postoperative catheterization, retained bladder clots, or recurrence of bleeding. The ultimate serious morbidity and mortality rates were comparably low, yet the patients of the faster surgeon recovered more rapidly at less total risk and cost.

Identification of these kinds of differences serves a variety of valuable functions. It has been shown repeatedly that physicians will respond to clinically valid information with self-correction.[4] Such differences are useful, therefore, in directed professional education, based on personal data. The department chair can motivate individual physician improvement by

Figure 6-1. Transurethral Resection Practice Indicators

1. Duration of procedures

2. Grams of tissue resected

3. ICU admission

4. Catheterized—days postop

5. Reinsertion of catheter

6. Readmission for bleeding, infection, or obstruction

7. Transfusion—units per case

8. Length of stay

9. Discharged with catheter

10. Death

11. Operative report on chart in 24 hours

Source: Adapted from Steven S. Lewis (personal communication, Yosemite, CA, 1988).

sharing clinically specific performance information in a confidential setting. This approach is more likely to modify physician behavior in a positive way than one that emphasizes restriction or limitation.

Purchasers of care and operators of health plans will also find these physician productivity profiles of value. Shorter lengths of stay and the use of fewer expensive ancillary services as a result of a "smoother" convalescence will identify such physicians as preferred providers. Presentation of such specific performance information during a contract negotiation can make the point that a given service gets better results and may be worth a higher per-unit price.

Adding several elements gleaned from the outpatient setting creates another important dimension. Hospitals that provide structured outpatient follow-up will be able to collect these data more easily. Those hospitals without organized outpatient programs will have difficulty obtaining this level of detail from independent physician offices. An independent practice association (IPA) or other hospital-related outpatient delivery system should have these data, however. These data are:

- Average total days of patient disability
- Total cost and ancillary service cost, inpatient and outpatient
- Mortality within 30 days of hospitalization
- Rate of degree of functional gain or loss

A reduced period of total disability followed by a full functional return translates into substantially less cost.

To meet the competitive needs of the 1990s, medical groups and hospitals will be obliged to demonstrate that their services meet these tests of cost-efficiency. Sophisticated buyers have already learned that price alone is not enough of a basis for differentiation. Much is said about quality as the next measure to be applied. Quality based solely on mortality or serious morbidity will prove to be insensitive to real service differences. The competitive edge will go to those physicians and hospitals whose patients return more predictably and more rapidly to full productive life. Not surprisingly, such patients are likely to cost less to insure.

One approach to differentiating the adequate from the good or great is to attempt, through data, to measure performance in a number of different ways. Using a procedure-specific approach, one can look at the goal of a particular procedure; its duration; the rate of success of achieving the goal; the rate of technique-related complications; the functional capacity of the patient at discharge; the frequency with which appliances, complex regimens, or repeat procedures are required; and so forth. These may be developed into a procedure-specific productivity profile.

Figures 6-2 through 6-11 list the generic and procedure-specific elements that may be considered in the development of *productivity practice*

Figure 6-2.   Generic Physician Productivity Indicators

Number of procedures

Outcome
   Status at discharge
   Total days of full disability
   Mortality rate 30 days posthospitalization

Time inputs
   Duration of procedure
   Number of days in intensive care
   Length of stay

Resource inputs
   Units of service, for example, specific laboratory test or X-ray studies per diagnosis or
      procedure

Success rate
   Estimate of functional gain or loss
   Patient satisfaction with result

Redo rate
   Cases with less than the desired outcome the first time requiring repetition

Error rate (after peer review)

Liability experience

Figure 6-3.   Cardiac Catheterization Practice Indicators

1. Fluoroscopy time

2. Number of injections

3. Volume of contrast media

4. Incomplete visualization of coronary vessels

5. Cardiac arrhythmia requiring drugs or cardioversion

6. Perforation of ventricle

7. Hematoma

8. Infection, puncture site or systemic

9. Myocardial infarction within 24 hours of procedure

10. Death

11. Cardiorespiratory arrest within 24 hours of procedure

12. Balloon angioplasty attempts

13. Emergency cardiac surgery directly from catheterization laboratory

14. Procedure report on chart within 24 hours

15. Second reader disagreement rate

16. Normal coronary circulation

Figure 6-4.   Bronchoscopy Practice Indicators

1. Duration of procedure
2. Visualization of organ expressed as a percentage
3. Biopsy—known lesion
4. Repeat study
5. Pneumothorax
6. Laryngeal injury
7. Successful termination of bleeding
8. Cardiorespiratory distress during or after procedure
9. Death within 24 hours
10. Normal examination
11. Procedure report on chart within 24 hours

Figure 6-5.   GI Endoscopy Practice Indicators

1. Duration of procedure
2. Visualization of organ expressed as percentage
3. Successful biopsy—known lesion
4. Repeat study
5. Perforation
6. Successful endoscopic retrograde visualization of the pancreatic duct
7. Successful termination of bleeding
8. Cardiorespiratory arrest
9. Death within 24 hours
10. Normal examination
11. Procedure report on chart within 24 hours

indicators. These may serve as the basis for procedure-specific performance indicators that could be incorporated in productivity profiles. Each department should be encouraged to develop similar sets covering their most common or most typical procedures. These should be individualized to suit physician interest and data-processing capability. For each institution or medical group, it will be necessary to validate these measures as surrogates of cost-efficient quality practice.

Procedures that are relatively standard and that are performed frequently lend themselves to this kind of analysis. The aim is to find at least one clinical activity per specialty that provides a quantitative measure of the physician's skill.

Note that the concept is applicable to invasive medical as well as common surgical procedures. As data sets used by insurance companies and self-insured employers improve, there will be a widespread use of similar evaluation schemes to identify "cheaper and better" physicians who will be the named preferred providers with whom payers will seek to contract.[5]

☐ Functional Status Evaluation

Functional status evaluation is likely to become an important tool in the assessment of medical interventions. Used initially in rehabilitation and cancer research, it has broader applicability. *Functional status* is a measure of the extent to which a patient has been returned to useful, meaningful life. It is applicable to both the employed and those who can no longer work. Functional status can be evaluated by the attending physician as part of the clinical examination. To illustrate, the goal of cataract surgery is to improve vision. Measurement of visual acuity before and several weeks after surgery should provide objective evidence of functional gain. Collection of these data provides the medical staff with one measure of how effective a given eye surgeon is.

☐ Peer Review and Productivity

Besides measuring physician effectiveness, the development of procedure-specific productivity profiles will be of value to the organized

Figure 6-6. Total Hip Replacement Practice Indicators

1. Description of adequate conservative trial

2. Description of joint pathology and functional limitation

3. Duration of surgery

4. Transfusion—during and after

5. Reoperation
   Cause—Infection
           Fracture
           Unstable prosthesis

6. Length of stay—in intensive care unit and in hospital
   Distance walked
   Discontinuation of analgesics

7. Ambulatory status with weight bearing at discharge and 2 weeks postdischarge

8. Death

9. Major medical complication

10. Operative report on chart in 24 hours

Figure 6-7. Abdominal Surgery Practice Indicators

1. Exploratory laparotomy

2. Negative exploration

3. Unplanned organ removal

4. Unplanned organ repair

5. Postoperative complication
    Hemorrhage
    Infection
    Intestinal obstruction
    Jaundice
    Fistula
    Wound dehiscence

6. Death

7. Unplanned ICU admission

8. Duration of procedure, elective transfusion, postoperative antibiotics, length of stay for the following procedures:
    Appendectomy
    Cholecystectomy
    Inguinal hernia
    Colon resection

9. Operative report on chart in 24 hours

---

medical staff or medical group for more typical credentialing and peer review purposes. Detailed tracking of physician performance over several years will eventually identify the physician with a declining trend. To illustrate, a skilled obstetrician can perform an emergency cesarean section in five to six minutes, measured from the time the anesthesiologist says "cut" to the time the infant is delivered. Any surgeon may be slowed by uterine fibroids or the adhesions of prior surgery. Yet if one determines the mean delivery time and plots it longitudinally for every case and for every department member, one can spot trends in the performance of this essential obstetrical service. If the trend indicates the obstetrician is slowing down, it provides a flag for more direct review. As a result, the medical staff has an opening for the exploration of personal attributes in the life of the physician. For example, the slowing may be caused by physical disability such as Parkinsonism or rheumatoid arthritis involving the hands and arms. Alternatively, the surgeon may be depressed for unrelated reasons or burned out by the stress of emergency obstetrics. In other circumstances, there may be self-treatment of an anxiety state with alcohol or benzodiazepines.

Supported by the data demonstrating decline in performance, the chief of staff or department chair can approach the physician. Sometimes that interaction alone will afford the obstetrician an opportunity to acknowledge a problem and turn to the medical staff for help. A referral at this point to a well-being or impaired-physician committee may be the first step toward recovery, if substance abuse or disability underlies the slow performance. Readers interested in more details about the relationship between physician health and medical staff privileges should consult *The Disabled Physician: Problem-Solving Strategies for the Medical Staff.*[6]

☐ Limitations of Profile Analysis

Statistical analyses and scorecards are no substitutes for careful physician review. Although we are fated to invest more resources to develop even more complex record systems, they will remain an adjunct to the basic peer review interaction. The following examples will make this point clear:

- A physician has an adverse result because of failure to recognize an obvious clinical condition and, therefore, effective treatment was omitted. This case is probably of sufficient seriousness to warrant some action without waiting for the two-year reappointment cycle to be up. Data in the physician's file may be helpful as background but the single case is sufficient for judgment.
- A surgeon has a perforated appendix rate of 25 percent. She has performed 20 procedures, in 5 of which a perforation was found at surgery. The departmental mean is 10 percent. A presumption is made that the surgeon is delaying surgery, perhaps by getting needless confirmatory tests before operating. The surgeon's ancillary service use is a bit higher than that of her peers. Individual case analysis, however,

Figure 6-8. Rhinoplasty Practice Indicators

1. Significant deformity or obstruction described
2. Relief of surgical indication
3. Transfusion
4. Reoperation
5. Cardiac arrhythmia
6. Airway infection—includes pneumonia
7. Endotracheal intubation, postoperative
8. Death
9. Operative report on chart in 24 hours
10. Preoperative and 6-week postoperative appearance comparison

Figure 6-9. Cesarean Section Indicators

Induction time (anesthesia to incision)

Delivery time (incision to delivery)

Total surgical time

Recovery time

Apgar 1/5 minutes

Transfusion
  Intraoperative
  Postoperative

Postop antibiotics—total days

Length of stay

Complications
  Maternal
  Fetal

Death
  Maternal
  Fetal

Justification

Rates
  Total primary C-sections
  Total C-sections
  Successful vaginal delivery after prior C-section
  Total unjustified C-sections after peer review

---

shows that four of the five patients are of an ethnic group known for stoicism and self-treatment. In each instance the patient was symptomatic for three days before contacting the surgeon.

- An obstetrician has a 10 percent seizure rate in the treatment of 30 patients with eclampsia. The mean for the department is a 1 percent seizure rate, and no other obstetrician has treated more than two patients with eclampsia. Quick analysis shows that the obstetrician is known as the department expert and sees all the serious preeclampsia patients in referral. The seizure rate is traced to two other members of the department who are slow to call for consultation.
- A pulmonologist has a mean length of stay for pneumonia of 10 days whereas the mean for the Department of Medicine is 6 days. Ancillary service use of X rays and antibiotics is correspondingly higher. Analysis shows that departmental statistics are skewed by several specialists in adolescent medicine who admit patients for four to five days for mycoplasma pneumonia. On the other hand, the pulmonologist sees elderly patients, often with mixed bacterial infection, who have failed treatment by other physicians.

Figure 6-10. Primary Care Practice Indicators

1. Admission after outpatient misadventure (for example, drug reaction, drug error)
2. Readmission after early discharge
3. Admission in advanced stage of disease
4. Unexpected death after medical staff review
5. Questioned drug or transfusion orders
6. Delayed or erroneous diagnosis
7. Unnecessary diagnostic admission
8. Discharge to a lower level of function or independence
9. Number and identity of consultants
10. Failure to respond to a key clinical value or test
11. Unavailable on call
12. Unwarranted delay of indicated surgery in inpatient
13. Adverse quality score assigned by Professional Standards Review Organization
14. Major medical record deficiencies
    a. Delayed or absent history and physical examination
    b. Delayed or absent discharge summary
    c. Absent progress notes

Figure 6-11. Perioperative Anesthesia Assessment

High block at or above 4th dorsal vertebra

Accidental spinal

Failed block

Drug reaction

Seizures

* Hypotension—< 80 min Hg systolic

* Hypertension—>160/90 min Hg

* Difficult intubation

* Aspiration

* Vomiting needing Rx

* Arrhythmia needing Rx

* Hypothermia < 95° F on entry into recovery room

* Hyperthermia >101° F

* Prolonged emergence from anesthetic

* To recovery room intubated

* To intensive care unit intubated

* Total recovery room time

* To be completed by recovery room nurse; the remainder by the responsible anesthesiologist

☐ Hazards of Aggregation

The preceding simple cases make clear the hazards of data aggregation without careful analysis. Coding either concurrently or retrospectively by record analysts is the usual basis for aggregation. Although coding practices are becoming more refined, there remains a significant error rate (10 percent in some studies). More important, the judgment of the coder is often incomplete. The perspective of the coder is to identify factors in a case that mandate assignment to a category with more or less similar cases. The physician, on the other hand, is obligated to distill from a case those unique elements that distinguish it from all others with the same or a similar diagnosis. Accuracy and fairness in peer review require analysis from the physician's point of view. Responsible peer review requires attention to details that might indicate specious aggregation, such as:

1. Risk factors such as age, stage of disease, comorbid conditions, severity, or acuity of presentation
2. The effect of prior treatment by other physicians for the same condition
3. The effect of concurrent treatment by other specialists for comorbid conditions
4. The unavoidable or rare complication
5. The actions of others on the treatment team, such as nurses or respiratory therapists
6. Independent patient factors such as cultural values, dietary traditions, noncompliance, and the like
7. The impact of utilization or payment schemes that may skew or limit management options

Even when one compares "apples to apples," it is necessary to recognize the difference between a small Granny Smith and a large Rome Beauty. Current profiling and aggregating schemes are inadequate to incorporate all of the significant individual factors that might influence a treatment decision or outcome. Coding and sorting systems to achieve that degree of specificity exist but are expensive. For peer review purposes, more detail in the sorting system leads to aggregation of fewer cases in each category. Research projects overcome this problem by the accrual of large numbers of cases in multiple centers. Systems like Medis-Groups or the data banks of the Professional Review Organizations accomplish the same thing. In the individual hospital, however, the number of cases will be too small for analysis, except case by case, for all but the most common procedures performed by the busiest practitioners. To overcome these problems, community hospitals aggregate cases that may be only superficially similar. Because of that, corrective action involving any limitation of clinical privileges must occur only after careful individual case review.

Review of a physician's credentials provides the medical staff with historical information on which to hazard an assignment of clinical privileges. It is at best an informed guess that in the usual setting is bolstered by initial concurrent proctoring to ensure the accuracy of the credentialing prediction. Satisfying that, the physician is monitored through the concurrent and retrospective screening mechanism of the quality assurance and peer review process. The goal of the aggregation of this information is not merely the accrual of a record of past cases, but also to provide the medical staff with a rational basis for deciding that the physician should be allowed to do the next case. Review, aggregation, analysis, and response by the medical staff, therefore, must be current and timely if that standard is to be met.

☐ Medical Staff Development Using the Physician Profile

Accrual of demographic information and its integration with the physician's practice pattern provides the basis for a tactical approach to medical staff development. Schlezinger[7] lists a number of elements to be tracked for the purpose of deciding which physicians should be courted, assisted, or shunned. These include:

- Inpatient and outpatient use/number of patients and trends
- Payer mix
- Cost of caring for patients
- Payment received for caring for patients, including percentage denied as outliers
- Consults requested by specialty and severity
- Consults given by specialty and severity
- Multiple staff membership—that is, the percentage referred to other hospitals
- Participation in medical staff activities
- Perception by members of hospital staff
- Perception by peers
- Overall quality of care
- Willingness to accept assistance
- Tenure on medical staff

Collecting this information permits an active, intelligent approach to medical staff development. Each physician must be evaluated as an individual to identify opportunities of mutual benefit. The medical staff planner must always be on the alert for physicians whose practices could be enhanced. The goal is to promote the interests of active effective physicians whose commitment to the hospital is clear. Less clear is the approach to the physician whose practice is counter to the interests of the hospital and the medical staff. Consistently poor quality, excessive utilization, and a predominance of patients whose coverage pays inadequately are all potential reasons why high volume is not enough to ensure a good relationship.

Although the peer review process must always remain the exclusive province of the medical staff, inevitably the conclusions drawn therefrom will find their way into the marketing and promotion activities regarding the hospital–medical staff delivery system. This is both appropriate and necessary. The reverse, the limitation of medical staff privileges for economic reasons, is an emerging battleground, to be discussed in the next chapter as part of the consideration of corrective action.

☐ References

1. Gosfield, A. G. Navigating through JCAH's new quality assurance and medical staff standards. *Healthspan* 4(2):3–9, Feb. 1987.

2. Schultz, R. Making computerized quality assurance work. *QRC Advisor* 6(8):1–8, June 1990.

3. Lewis, S. Personal communication, Yosemite, CA, 1988.

4. Eisenberg, J. M. Doctors' decisions and the cost of medical care. *Health Administration Press Perspectives.* Ann Arbor, MI: Health Administration Press, 1986.

5. Robinson, M. L. Huge Medicare files to back outcomes research. *Hospitals* 62(16):18, Aug. 20, 1988.

6. Lang, D. A., Jara, G. B., and Kessenick, L. W. *The Disabled Physician: Problem-Solving Strategies for the Medical Staff.* Chicago: American Hospital Publishing, 1989.

7. Schlezinger, I. H. (Hillcrest Medical Center, Tulsa, OK). Presentation at American Hospital Association Convention, July 30, 1990 [as cited in the *Medical Executive Committee Reporter,* Sept. 1990, published by the National Health Foundation].

Chapter 7

Corrective Action

If the goal of peer review is the defense of medical staff standards in the interest of continuous quality improvement, it follows then that corrective action is its measure of effectiveness. Collecting data and identifying outliers are not enough. Using the information to effect change is the true te꜀ ꜀f medical staff skill and courage. Absent thoughtful corrective action, ꜀. ꜀rything else is a meaningless and costly process. Peer review is worth the price only if the medical staff imparts value to it through appropriate use.

Medical staffs characteristically have difficulty with the application of corrective action. Analysis of medical staff responses to problem cases will be helpful in understanding the reasons for this. On the basis of extensive review of medical staff minutes and discussions with physicians, the author finds that medical staffs initially respond to a clinical performance problem in the following ways (in increasing order of intrusiveness):

- Collecting data passively—keeping track without informing the physician
- Soliciting additional information from the physician
- Writing to the physician about medical staff standards without identifying the patient or the specific breach of standards
- Organizing a program of continuing medical education without identifying the patient
- Sending a letter to the physician in which the specific clinical problem is identified and alternative medical staff management is suggested

Usually when the medical staff elects the passive or more diffident response, it does so in response to one of several concerns:

1. Identification of the patient will violate confidentiality of peer review, and the error will become discoverable in a professional liability action.

2. A diffident, respected approach is one that does not imply the physician did anything wrong. It sends a vague message that there *might have been* a problem.

3. General continuing medical education is sufficient to effect change somehow, even if the physician with the problem case doesn't attend.

4. Avoiding the confrontation implied by identifying the patient and the breach of standards reduces the risk of physician backlash including suits for defamation, bias, and anticompetitive action.

5. As peer review is an offensive responsibility imposed from without, the least intrusive response that gets by is sufficient.

6. Paradoxically, one may also see an inappropriately harsh response from inexperienced medical staffs. For example, a physician will have a series of cases fall out of quality assurance screening. Several will be referred for departmental review, which might find a rule infraction and perhaps a complication. The medical staff takes this set of circumstances as justification for a summary suspension of the physician's privileges "to show how tough and decisive we can be" or "to set an example for others." Valid reasons exist for summary deprivation of a physician's privileges, but "medical staff machismo" is not one of them.

From these examples, then, it is evident that identification of an outlier or problem case elicits a complex emotional response in both the reviewed physician and the reviewer. The situation is more emotional the more it is ad hoc. The challenge for the medical staff is to develop a policy that recognizes nuances and to tailor the medical staff's response to the problems of the physician whose care is under question, while at the same time maintaining consistency and fairness. One must bear in mind constantly that the goal of corrective action is the modification of physician behavior in the interests of patient safety. To achieve this end, the medical staff must design an approach to corrective action that is specific and individualized, and yet consistent and fair.

☐ Range of Corrective Actions Permitted by Bylaws

All corrective action strategies must be based on authority granted the medical staff by its bylaws. The following list of corrective action options for modification of physician behavior is available to virtually all medical staffs:

- Education
- Positive incentives
- Focused education—identified problem
- Concurrent monitoring—direct investigative observation
- Mandatory second opinion—preprocedure
- Mandatory presence of a qualified second physician

- Temporary loss of privileges
- Partial permanent loss of privileges
- Suspension of membership
- Dismissal or revocation
- Denial of reappointment
- Denial of appointment after provisional year
- Denial of active status after leave of absence

The range of possible actions extends from the general and positive to the very specific and restrictive. Medical staffs may be creative in tailoring individual corrective action programs within these broad categories.

☐ A Graded Approach to Corrective Action

Table 7-1 presents a classification of diagnostic errors found at autopsy.[1] Note that they range from imperfect medical knowledge to "willful or malicious error." This type of observation provides the theoretical basis for the concept of graded corrective action, detailed in table 7-2.

Table 7-1. Types of Diagnostic Errors by Etiology

Category	Type of Error	Definition
A	Imperfect medical knowledge	Unavoidable errors due to limitations in current medical knowledge
B	Necessary fallibility	Unavoidable errors caused by the unpredictability in a specific patient–physician interaction
C	Practitioner error	Errors due to limitations in the knowledge or skills of the physician
D	Willful or malicious error	Negligent or willful disregard of accepted norms

Source: Reprinted, with permission, from Anderson, R. E. How autopsy can be used in quality assessment. *QA Review* 1(4), Nov. 1989.

Table 7-2. Graded Corrective Action

Performance Element	Corrective Action	Due Process Protection
Knowledge deficit	Focused education	Informal review; letter of admonition
Skill deficit	Focused training	Same as above, plus proctoring
Temporary loss of capacity	Physical and mental evaluation Adjusted privileges	Physician aid Fair hearing Monitoring contract
Inability to change	Restriction/dismissal	Fair hearing

Focused Education and Training

According to the concept of graded corrective action, if a clinical event is judged to be the result of a knowledge deficit, the appropriate medical staff response would be to take focused education. Examples of focused education include:

- A general education program such as grand rounds based on a specific case or problem, where there is a lesson for the staff as a whole.
- Presentation at a department meeting.
- A letter to the physician outlining the specific event and the appropriate way of avoidance. For example, the letter might describe a patient who had a heart block due to a failure of the attending physician to withhold the digitalis glycoside when the patient exhibited warning signs of vomiting and premature heartbeats.
- A letter of admonition or warning describing the possibility of restriction or other sanction if a given problem or practice recurs. This approach intensifies the educational experience by the contemplation of more drastic action.
- Focused mandatory tutoring in which the physician is required to meet with a medical staff specialist for instruction in a specific area of knowledge deficiency. If this option is used, the date, time, and content summary of the tutorial should be reported in the department minutes.
- Mandatory formal education such as requiring six hours of continuing medical education in the use of antibiotics where a physician has had problems in their appropriate use. In unusual instances where there is evidence of a significant knowledge gap, this might require a return to a formal training program. Evidence of successful completion would be required.

Similar principles apply if the physician exhibits a deficiency in performing technical skills, in which case the educational or training efforts would be focused on the specific deficit. Demonstration of mastery of the skill, as attested to by the trainer and by medical staff proctoring, would be required (see chapter 3 for more on proctoring).

Physician and Mental Evaluation/Adjusted Privileges

If a clinical event is judged to be attributable to a loss of physician capacity, the medical staff must determine whether the loss is temporary or permanent. This entails a physical and mental examination of the physician as well as an analysis of performance records. Depending on the severity of the problem exhibited, the medical staff might consider temporary or summary suspension of the physician's privileges. Consider, for example, a diabetic physician who has had a series of insulin reactions and was unable to complete a surgery. That physician might be temporarily suspended, pending regulation of diabetes. On the other hand, a surgeon who was unable to complete a procedure because of drunkenness or psychotic behavior would be considered for a summary suspension of privileges.

Summary Suspension

Bylaws usually allow for a summary suspension of medical staff privileges when the actions of a physician constitute an immediate threat to the health or safety of a patient, hospital employee, physician, or visitor. This is usually interpreted to mean that as a result of observations of the physician's behavior or quality of care, he or she is judged to be unfit to exercise previously granted privileges, and they are abruptly terminated.

One occasionally sees a bylaws provision that allows for temporary suspension while a physician is being investigated for clinical problems indicative of a loss of professional skills. If the patient risk is serious, the suspension may be justified. The danger, of course, in either temporary or summary suspension is that the argument regarding the physician shifts from the question of clinical competence to that of the appropriateness (according to the bylaws) of the abrupt removal of privileges. Bylaws requirements for accelerated review by the Executive Committee and a fair hearing compress the time for the medical staff to prepare its case. Many a medical staff has learned the hard way that a case that warranted some restriction of a physician was ultimately shown to be insufficient for summary suspension.

In either event, the physician would be entitled to a formal medical staff hearing and appeal regarding the appropriateness of the suspension. Where illness was a factor, the physician would also have to show some evidence of a return to health before privileges were restored. Execution of a monitoring agreement, in which the physician agreed to submit to random mandatory neurophysiologic and biochemical testing, would be required as a condition for retaining privileges. For a more detailed discussion of the management of this situation, see *The Disabled Physician.*[2]

A physician may be judged to be unable to respond to the supportive efforts of the medical staff. This judgment may be arrived at as a consequence of the following:

- Failure to submit to mandated education or training
- Failure to participate in mandated reviews of questioned patient care

- Failure to undergo treatment or rehabilitation for identified physical or mental problems, including substance abuse
- Failure to show adherence to rehabilitation programs as manifested by inability to pass random mandatory neurophysiologic or biochemical testing
- Performance of a case or a series of cases that exhibit gross and flagrant negligence to a degree indicative of major loss of professional skill or judgment

☐ Severity Grades for Adverse Events

The medical staff, in applying these general principles of corrective action, may be guided by a system that promises to minimize inconsistencies or unwarranted extremes of medical staff response. A grading system based on the severity of the clinical event and the degree of physician culpability is presented in figure 7-1. Records that fall out of screening, after final department review, are assigned a grade in ascending order of severity from the perspective of the medical staff. An example of grade 1 might be a case in which a patient with known coronary artery disease developed transient angina following an indicated procedure. Grade 2 would be assigned if that same patient had transient ischemic EKG changes because the physician failed to reorder nitroglycerin or because the procedures ordered were unexpectedly too taxing. Grade 3 would apply if that same patient sustained serious myocardial ischemia requiring ICU admission and angioplasty, but had no significant loss of myocardial tissue. Grade 4 would result if the patient had a major myocardial infarction. Grade 5 would result if death was the outcome. Grade 6 would apply if the physician was unavailable or failed to recognize the complication because of inattention. Similarly, grade 6 might result if the taxing procedures were clearly unwarranted or ordered or

Figure 7-1. Severity Grades: Adverse Events

Grade 1. A minor error or complication with no injury, cause not attributable

Grade 2. A minor error or complication with injury with no disability or treatment change, caused by physician omission or commission

Grade 3. A major error or complication with no disability but requiring major treatment change (such as ICU or emergency surgery), caused by physician omission or commission

Grade 4. A major error or complication with permanent disability or injury evident at time of hospital discharge, caused by physician omission or commission

Grade 5. A major error or complication leading to death, caused by physician omission or commission

Grade 6. Any grade 3, 4, or 5 event caused by gross negligence performed in the face of clear warnings by consultants to avoid them. Grade 6 severity would also be considered if the procedures were performed over the express objections of the patient.

Medical Staff Response by Severity of Event

Figure 7-2 lists the medical staff corrective action responses in ascending order of severity of effect on the physician's practice. The corrective action response takes into consideration a number of components, all of which must be considered as part of the process.

By combining the concepts of graded severity of event and generic response, as presented in figures 7-1 and 7-2, it is possible to standardize the corrective action measures that are available to the medical staff in a given situation. Figure 7-3 presents a system whereby more serious adverse events lead to more stringent medical staff actions. These actions range from informal communication with the physician, recorded in departmental quality assurance and peer review records or minutes, to summary removal of a physician's privileges to practice.

Figure 7-2. Components of Corrective Action

Communication with physician
- Verbal or written
- General or patient-specific
- Instruction, admonition, or warning

Notation of review and communication
- On the worksheet
- In the minutes of the Peer Review Committee
- In the physician's credential or quality assurance file

Prospective evaluation of physician's skill, knowledge, or capacity
- Investigational proctoring
- Postdischarge record review
*• Mandatory consultation
*• Mandatory comanagement
*• Random mandatory neurophysiologic and biochemical testing

Limitation of the physician's privileges
- Reduction of privileges to eliminate more complicated or riskier ones
- Elimination of all medical staff privileges

Phase-in of limitation
- Temporary suspension pending investigation
- Summary suspension
- Denial of reappointment
- Limitation recommended by Executive Committee without restriction, pending hearing and appeal

*These are also considered limitations of the physician's privileges.

Figure 7-3.   Medical Staff Response by Severity of Event

Grade 1.   Informal discussion with physician with notation on review form or worksheet.

Grade 2.   Informal discussion or letter to physician, either action noted in the minutes of the Peer Review Committee or the department data base and logged in the QA file of physician.

Grade 3.   Letter of admonition or warning to physician noted in minutes, inserted into credentials file, and logged in QA file. Consider limitation or restriction if repeat event. Investigational proctoring prior to final decision.

Grade 4.   Letter of admonition or warning noted in minutes, inserted in credentials file, and logged in QA file. Limitation or restriction such as mandatory second opinion or consultation. Investigational proctoring prior to final decision.

Grade 5.   Letter of inquiry to physician. Response noted in committee minutes, credentials file, and QA file. Investigational proctoring prior to final decision. Limitation or restriction such as loss of privileges likely.

Grade 6.   Summary restriction or suspension.

Grounds for Dismissal or Denial of Reappointment

Medical staffs may gain further consistency and confidence in the application of corrective action by identifying thresholds for action. As an extension of the grading schemes in figures 7-1, 7-2, and 7-3, further clarity might result from the medical staff's contemplation of (in the abstract) and answer to the following question: "What does it take to be dismissed from or denied reappointment to our medical staff?" Figure 7-4 presents 10 screening criteria to guide reappointment. These criteria are based on data ordinarily collected or available for medical staff review. Failure to meet any of these criteria would mandate special medical staff review prior to reappointment. Failure to meet any of criteria numbers 4 through

Figure 7-4.   Screening Criteria to Guide Reappointment

1. Sufficient utilization to allow assurance of clinical competence

2. Cases admitted or performed consistent with privileges requested

3. Cases admitted or performed reviewed by quality assurance peer review

4. No cases identified that have led to suspension or loss of privileges for poor-quality care

5. No convictions for felonies, reimbursement fraud, or clinical negligence

6. No evidence of deterioration in health severe enough to impair clinical privileges

7. Office and/or residence close enough to permit prompt response

8. Professional liability cases reveal no pattern of negligent or incompetent care

9. Lost membership or privileges in other hospitals, clinics, or professional organizations reveal no pattern of negligent or incompetent care

10. No restriction of license or certification for disciplinary reasons

10 would require special justification to permit reappointment. Any physician would be considered for dismissal if—either at the time of reappointment or after—he or she exhibited any of the following:

- Persistent failure of performance
- Serious loss of professional skill
- Serious loss of physical or mental skills
- Gross personal negligence
- Conviction of felonies involving fraud, violence, or careless disregard for human safety
- Loss of license to practice
- Failure to meet requirements of the medical staff for meeting attendance, liability insurance, emergency call panel backup, timely and accurate completion of medical records, and so forth

Each medical staff may differ in how it defines terms such as *persistent, serious,* or *gross.* The point of the exercise of definition is to establish for the medical staff a behavioral standard that can be cited when a specific problem physician is identified.

For example, consider a psychiatrist who has a series of patients who come to harm or who die after admission because of a persistent failure to recognize them as suicide risks and to order appropriate precautions. This unfortunate sequence continues despite peer review and counseling. The medical staff would be justified to conclude, based on a pattern of substandard care that persisted after counseling and warning, that the physician demonstrated a persistent failure of performance. Dismissal is then warranted, either after medical staff hearing or by denial of reappointment.

☐ Economic Credentialing

Medical staffs and hospitals are under increasing pressure to improve the efficiency with which care is rendered. It is tempting to set performance goals and then apply sanctions when they are not met. This is undoubtedly an extension of the industrial model that mandates so many widgets per hour as a criterion for employment or reward. This simplistic approach is inappropriate for the medical staff, even if modified to reflect only length of stay, resource use, or review agency denial rates.[3] Yet it is possible to develop a strategy of information and graded intervention that may help modify the individual physician's practice pattern in the direction of enhanced efficiency. The strategy should incorporate the following elements:

1. Collection of data comparing performance of the individual physician to the medical staff as a whole regarding the following:

- Length of stay.
- Resource use (X rays, MRI, ICU days, antibiotics, and so on) by DRG or other homogeneous diagnostic category.
- Productivity as measured by mean duration of common standard procedures, redo rates, error rates after peer review, and so on.

2. Assessment of physician's performance as evaluated by review agencies, including:
   - Medical staff utilization review and quality assurance or departmental committee's denial or adverse judgment rate.
   - External agency (PRO, Medicaid) denial rate.
   - Internal and external appeals rejected.
   - Internal or external sanctions.

3. Provision in the medical staff bylaws of graded action options, such as:
   - Education, general and focused on the individual physician.
   - Development of physician-specific economic performance profiles (see the first element in this list).
   - Initiation of quality assurance evaluation and/or peer review triggered by economic flags such as resource use and length of stay.
   - Consideration of criteria for loss of right to participate in the medical staff independent practice association, to receive patients from the hospital's referral service, or to practice on the backup panel of the emergency department.

     These criteria might include unjustified economic loss because of a pattern of failure to practice within requirements of various managed care programs, including Medicare and Medicaid, after independent evaluation by the medical staff. Another criterion might be the failure to refer to the hospital cases that arise from the hospital's referral or call panels, where hospitalization is required and the institution is adequate for the clinical problem.
   - Denial of reappointment where there has been an unjustified pattern of inefficient practice after repeated warnings and resistance to behavioral change, especially where it is possible to show an adverse effect of economic loss on the care and resources available to other patients. Obviously, this is an extreme measure, to be attempted infrequently and with great thought and preparation.

4. Discussion of resource use with the physician. Armed with good information and the authority to use it, the chief of staff or medical director discusses resource use with the attending physician. A strong pitch is made to improve economic performance.

□ Mitigation of Corrective Action by Reporting Requirements

The advent of the National Practitioner Data Bank will bring to the national scene a paradoxical phenomenon observed in states that have had physician disciplinary reporting requirements. Any restriction or limitation of a physician's privileges to practice, including denial of membership in an organized medical staff or professional society, must be reported to the centralized agency (see chapter 8 for more on the data bank).[4] Physicians in states with similar reporting requirements and data banks have sought to tailor medical staff action to just below the threshold of required reporting. Where any discipline-related change of status had to be reported, physicians facing discipline negotiated resignations in lieu of reports. This led to a requirement to report resignations or withdrawals in anticipation of investigation or discipline. Some boards have considered a requirement to report any change of privilege regardless of cause.

The net result of these requirements is an emphasis on education and admonition without privilege limitation. One can legitimately hold that given the nature of most cases, that is all that is warranted. Certainly the principles articulated above would lead to a conclusion that the first efforts at corrective action should be educational or nonrestrictive, especially under circumstances where there was no major disability caused nor gross negligence.

Physicians have come to regard the reporting of disciplinary action to a government agency as an added punishment. In California, this has led to legislation, SB1211, which mandates a full judicial hearing and appeal process for any physician subjected to a medical staff action that is reportable to the state licensure board. The paradox, of course, is that physicians are averse to entering the name of a colleague into a government computer. Medical staffs, therefore, are more likely to avoid taking corrective action that mandates such reporting. Absent the need for reporting of limitation, the likelihood is that medical staffs would impose more mandatory second opinions and consultations. At present, most authorities hold that investigational proctoring, imposed as part of the evaluation of a case before final action, is not reportable. Some authorities close to the National Practitioner Data Bank prefer that proctoring in that context be reportable, even though patient care may be appropriate and no limitation of privileges eventuates. If history is any guide, should investigational proctoring become reportable, medical staffs will avoid the use of this essential tool as well.

Unfortunately, this conflict about the threshold of reportability of medical staff action misses the point. Determinants of medical staff corrective action should be the nature of the offense, its effect on the patient, the existence of a pattern of prior offenses, and the effect of prior efforts at education or rehabilitation. The medical staff action should not be determined by its desire to report or avoid reporting to the National Practitioner Data Bank. Such reporting should follow where discipline or restriction resulted from a decision based on the determinants listed previously. Failure of the medical staff to take forthright action to avoid reporting places it in the role of protector of a physician whose level of practice may not warrant protection. Such failure may send a signal that, regardless of the circumstances, the medical staff is afraid to take effective corrective action either because of misplaced compassion or fear of retribution triggered by the report. Whereas state statutes exempt physicians from liability for the act of reporting, they do not protect adequately against allegations of harassment, bias, and defamation during the investigation or hearing that leads to the report.

References

1. Anderson, R. E. How autopsy can be used in quality assessment. *QA Review* 1(4), Nov. 1989.
2. Lang, D. A., Jara, G. B., and Kessenick, L. W. *The Disabled Physician: Problem-Solving Strategies for the Medical Staff.* Chicago: American Hospital Publishing, 1989.
3. Berwick, D. M. Continuous improvement as an ideal in health care. *New England Journal of Medicine* 320(1):53, Jan. 5, 1989.
4. U.S. Department of Health and Human Services, Public Health Service, Health Resources and Services Administration. *National Practitioner Data Bank Guidebook.* Washington, DC: USDHHS, 1990.

Chapter 8

An Overview of Current Legal Issues in Peer Review

Corrective action can be effective only if it is sustainable. Nothing so frustrates the peer review activity of the medical staff as the rejection of one of its decisions on the grounds that the processes it used were flawed or the actions unwarranted. Rejection of a judgment of the medical staff to remove or limit a physician's privileges calls into question all of the effort expended. "Why bother? It's not worth the risk or the hassle" is the usual response. Consequently, participation in the next peer review action is harder to achieve.

Worse, in this litigious era, every peer review action carries with it the threat of a counteraction in the courts by the reviewed physician. It doesn't matter whether the medical staff prevailed in its internal review and appeals. If the limitation on the physician stands, he or she is likely to sue to attempt to overturn it. If the limitation is rejected by the medical staff or governing body appeals process, the physician, rather than simply being relieved, is likely to sue on the grounds that exoneration proves that the original peer review action was taken for base reasons. Unjustified defamation, libel, slander, or emotional injury is likely to be alleged.

Small wonder, then, that the physician who participates in peer review feels he or she can't win. Yet, in the interests of professional responsibility and improvement of patient care, physicians do persist in peer review. With the risks of success or failure so high, that persistence is warranted only if review is carried out in a manner that withstands the almost inevitable challenge. To do that, every step taken must conform to the requirements of fair process, as outlined in the medical staff bylaws, statutes, and applicable court decisions. A detailed legal analysis of this process is beyond the scope of this book. For a detailed practical approach to the fair hearing, see Liset.[1] For a more precise application of the law to particular events, legal counsel should be sought.

The goal of this chapter is to identify common problems physicians and hospitals face in peer review and corrective action and to suggest ways of avoiding them. A question-and-answer format will be used to focus on typical physician and administration concerns in the peer review process.

Q. *What is the legal authority for peer review?*

A. Physicians reviewing the work of other physicians is a hallowed professional tradition arising out of clinical care conferences in dim historical times. Its value as a method for improving patient care has been recognized in regulation and statute. Hospital licensure statutes require the medical staff to engage in peer review. Payment for Medicare under "Conditions of Participation" (COP) is possible only in hospitals whose medical staffs have an effective review process. For a detailed interpretation of Medicare COP, see the 1990 Institute of Medicine analysis.[2] Accreditation by the JCAHO also requires "monitoring and evaluation" of patient care.[3]

Q. *Why does the physician submit to peer review?*

A. The physician accepts the provisions of the medical staff bylaws when applying for membership. Adherence to these bylaws is the price paid for the privilege to practice in the hospital. Medical staff bylaws provide that care will be reviewed. The mechanisms of that peer review are detailed, as is the range of options for corrective action and the rights of the physician to appeal those actions.

Q. *What is the usual basis for corrective action?*

A. On review of a case or a series of cases performed by the physician, the medical staff judges that the professional care rendered was below the hospital's standards of practice. Although the trigger for review may be a numerical standard, such as a high complication rate or high mortality rate, the basis for corrective action will be physician failure to follow professional standards, causing the adverse result, as demonstrated by specific cases. The burden of proof for the medical staff is demonstration of that professional failure. Basing corrective action on specific cases and actions, in fairness, allows the physician to provide information in defense or mitigation.

Q. *What procedures does the medical staff follow in corrective action?*

A. The usual process has the following elements:
- Recognition by the clinical department that the physician's privileges should be limited.
- Request in writing by the department to the Medical Executive Committee (MEC) for limitation. At times, the MEC will initiate the review and limitation on its own.
- An informal interview to allow the physician to present his or her side of the story to the MEC. Minutes of the interview are kept

as a basis for further action and future reference. As Liset[4] points out, an interview at this point allows the medical staff to discover the physician's reasoning, as he or she may be held to that reasoning in subsequent proceedings.

- Affirmation of the decision to limit privileges to a degree consistent with the problem identified. For example, if a surgeon demonstrates loss of manual skill, operating room privileges may be removed whereas admitting and consultation privileges will remain intact. The goal of the limitation is the protection of patient safety, although protection of the hospital, other professionals, or the physicians in question may be legitimate secondary goals.
- Written communication to the physician detailing the limitation and informing him or her of the right to appeal. A copy of the bylaws with the appeal process highlighted may be provided at this time.

Q. *How does the physician appeal the limitation of privileges?*

A. Medical staff bylaws provide for a fair hearing plan that outlines the appeals procedure, which usually is initiated by the physician's written request within time frames spelled out in the bylaws.

Q. *What are the essential elements of the medical staff appeal process?*

A. These may vary but most bylaws have certain elements in common. Commonality has been enhanced by the Health Care Quality Improvement Act (HCQIA) of 1986,[5] which established federal guidelines for fair hearings as a safe haven from accusation of antitrust violation. In some states (California, for example) these steps fall under statutory regulations as well.

- In response to a request for a fair hearing, a written statement of charges to the physician is prepared, spelling out in detail the specific cases and the specific failings on which the corrective action is based. This is usually prepared by the hospital's attorney using factual information provided by the medical executive committee. This is usually sent by certified mail.
- A hearing date is set at least 30 days after the charges are received.
- A listing of prehearing rights may be furnished to the physician. These rights include:
  - Discovery
  - Attorney assistance in case preparation (although HCQIA 1986 requires participation by the physician's attorney in the hearing for maximum protection from an antitrust allegation)
  - Continuance for cause
  - Receipt of witness list
- Formal or judicial hearing rights, including:
  - An impartial panel including the right to challenge the panel members or the hearing officer on the grounds of bias or conflict of interest (voir dire)

- Evidence examination
- Presentation of witnesses and rebuttal testimony
- Attorney representation during the hearing
- A written summary of the findings of the hearing and the basis for the decision

Q. *What is the standard of proof in the hearing?*

A. The Hearing Committee may use information (including hearsay) to arrive at a judgment based on a preponderance of evidence. A nexus between the events in question and the quality of patient care must be shown by the peer review body of the medical staff.

Q. *Does the physician whose care is questioned have the right to further appeal?*

A. The HCQIA and most medical staff bylaws provide for the right of the accused physician to appeal to the governing body of the hospital. The appeal must be in writing. It generally is based on the assertion that the decision was in error or the process of arriving at it was flawed.

Q. *Why should medical staffs follow the guidelines of the HCQIA?*

A. The HCQIA was passed as a consequence of the demonstration in *Patrick v. Burget*[6] that anticompetitive motivation could underlie peer review actions. In that decision, it was judged that the basis for removing the physician from his medical staff was not purely in the interests of patient safety but rather (perhaps primarily) to get rid of a competitor in a small community. Without going into detail, the processes employed by the medical staff did not provide Patrick sufficient protection. The congressional response to *Patrick* was the HCQIA, which established guidelines for the peer review process, which have been incorporated in the foregoing material. Adhering to these guidelines will protect the medical staff against challenges of unfairness of its processes. Strict application of HCQIA guidelines provides a safe harbor from the allegation that federal antitrust statutes were violated in bringing the peer review action.

Under the HCQIA, a peer review body must have met the following conditions to qualify for immunity:

(1) It acted in the reasonable belief that the action was in the furtherance of quality health care.

(2) It acted after a reasonable effort to obtain the facts of the matter.

(3) It acted only after adequate notice and hearing procedures were afforded the physician or after such other procedures as were fair to the physician under the circumstances.

(4) It acted in the reasonable belief that the action was warranted by the facts known after such reasonable effort to obtain facts and after meeting the requirement of paragraph (3).

Note that the HCQIA does not protect against allegations that the peer review action was a violation of the physician's civil rights because of race, sex, national origin, or political belief. In a recent case (*Austin v. Santa Barbara College Hospital, et al.*),[7] the HCQIA has been held to provide antitrust immunity if the guidelines are followed.

Q. *If a physician serves on a Peer Review Committee, can he or she be sued?*[8,9]

A. Physicians who serve on peer review committees run the risk of being sued for the following reasons:
- The peer reviewer acted out of malice.
- There was an economic conflict of interest in which the peer reviewer benefited from the physician's restriction.
- The actions of the peer reviewer were the result of an anticompetitive conspiracy.
- There was bias because of age, race, sex, national origin, or professional training.
- There was a deliberate and substantive breach of process.

  Although a peer reviewer is always a potential suit victim, the likelihood may be minimized by the following approach:
- If simply screening the record for further committee review, be objective and follow the medical staff standards that mandate referral.
- The Peer Review Committee or department that receives referred records from the screening physician should be made up of physicians who are not direct competitors, although they may be in the same specialty or clinical department.
- The Peer Review Committee or department has no authority to restrict, although it may formally warn or reprimand.
- Restriction of a physician's privileges (except for summary suspension) should occur only after deliberation by the Medical Executive Committee which, in all but single-specialty hospitals, will be composed of physicians from a variety of noncompeting areas of practice.
- Where a physician is summarily suspended, the suspension must be promptly reviewed by the Medical Executive Committee to ensure that it was warranted. The usual basis is that summary suspension was necessary to avoid immediate risk of harm to a patient, hospital employee, or others because of improper and otherwise uncontrollable actions of the physician. Because summary suspension seriously limits the physician, and thus carries with it the burden of prompt justification and review, it also carries with it a higher likelihood of litigation. The safest standard on which to base a summary suspension is the clear and immediate danger of harm by the physician to another person.
- Physicians who serve on a Judicial Review or Appeals Committee should not have participated in the decision to limit the

physician-appellant. As well, they should have no bias or malice and must gain no competitive advantage from a decision to restrict or limit.

Q. *What are the hazards for the physician who refuses to participate in the peer review process?*

A. In a single case, there may be none. According to most medical staff bylaws, however, a repeated pattern of refusal to participate can lead to reduction in medical staff status, from attending physician to courtesy. Loss of medical staff privileges, in most instances, is unlikely.

Q. *What are the risks if the entire medical staff refuses to participate in the peer review process?*

A. If the hospital is sued for malpractice in which physician competence is at issue, there may be added liability if the peer review process is inadequate.[10-12]

- If there is general knowledge about an incompetent physician and the peer review body fails to deal with it, the peer review body may be sued on grounds of a "conspiracy of silence." The hospital would bear the liability for such an action in a subsequent malpractice action. Both the medical staff and the hospital would suffer from the attendant adverse publicity.

- Failure to perform effective or meaningful peer review is grounds for citation if not revocation of hospital licensure, accreditation,[13] and certification for payment as a Medicare provider.

Q. *Is the physician who participates in peer review protected by the hospital?*[14]

A. Most hospitals provide insurance coverage for physicians who participate in the review of their peers. This insurance generally covers all actions taken by physicians as part of the formal medical staff processes. To ensure protection, authority for the action must be defined in the medical staff bylaws and rules and regulations. Communication about cases under review should take place only during regularly constituted medical staff committee meetings. If informal or ad hoc meetings are convened to deal with a matter, they should be authorized by a committee and their results reported back. These precautions also ensure maximum confidentiality of committee deliberations. Insurance coverage does not usually extend to payment of awards or settlements for actions based on antitrust, bias, or malice. The defense of such suits is generally provided but, unless the physician is employed by the hospital, indemnification is counter to public policy.

The best protection for the physician reviewer comes from adherence to the processes outlined in a well-designed set of medical staff bylaws or regulations. Training in the provisions of these bylaws and rules minimizes the risk of inadvertent error. Adequate legal support is a must to guide the process, especially as states are likely to differ in their individual requirements.

Q. *What is the National Practitioner Data Bank, and how does it relate to the peer review process?*

A. The National Practitioner Data Bank was established as a provision of HCQIA. The National Practitioner Data Bank requires that hospitals, professional societies, physician groups, and "other health care entities" report adverse actions lasting more than 30 days against clinical privileges or membership of a physician based on professional competence. Malpractice settlements or judgments resulting in any payment and adverse actions by a state licensure board must also be reported. Hospitals must query the National Practitioner Data Bank on initial appointment and at least every two years as part of its privilege-granting process for each member of its medical staff. Data received are designed to alert the hospital if the physician had problems in professional competence in other hospitals in the country. Hospitals and other entities that fail to report will be subject to substantial fine or loss of immunity under Title IV of the HCQIA. If a hospital fails to request information about a physician as required, it may be presumed to have known about adverse information in the file. A plaintiff or plaintiff's attorney, then, can petition the Department of Health and Human Services (HHS) for access to the physician's National Practitioner Data Bank file for use in a malpractice action against the hospital and the physician. A physician may query the bank about his or her own file at any time, free of charge.

The National Practitioner Data Bank began collecting information and issuing reports on September 1, 1990. Information, once entered, can be revised only on appeal to the secretary of HHS. Medical staffs should establish a protocol for review of any proposed report with the involved physician to ensure agreement on the accuracy of the information prior to submission. The time for submission of reports of limitation or withdrawal of physician privileges is 15 days from the date the order to limit or withdraw is signed by the responsible hospital official, even if the action is under appeal. Presumably, if the action does not commence until after all internal appeals are exhausted, reporting would be deferred until that point. Voluntary relinquishing of privileges while under investigation for a matter of professional competence or discipline is reportable as well.

Requirements to report will undoubtedly lead medical staffs to limit corrective actions to those that need not be reported, such as letters of reprimand, suspensions of less than 30 days, and investigational proctoring. They are likely to lead to the development of precise training and experience standards for the granting of privileges. Failure to meet these standards on the face is not a matter of professional competence or discipline, per se. This is obviously a gray area, and case law ultimately will define more sharply what must be reported.

The National Practitioner Data Bank must be queried for all physicians, including those applying for temporary privileges. Some hospitals have elected to defer granting temporary privileges until the National Practitioner Data Bank has replied to a request for information. Others have granted temporary privileges pending the report. A few hospitals no longer grant temporary privileges at all.

National Practitioner Data Bank regulations are detailed and complex. This summary only skims the surface. A toll-free Data Bank Help Line (1-800/767-6732) is available to answer questions. Individual hospitals should review their protocols with their attorneys to ensure full compliance.

Q. *How can antitrust or anticompetitive lawsuits be avoided in small hospitals or small clinical departments?*

A. In small facilities, especially in rural communities, the impact of the restriction of one physician is likely to be felt by all others involved. The risk of challenge that the action is motivated by personal gain is real and may be difficult to disprove. Nonetheless, this possibility does not relieve the small medical staff from its review obligations. Standards setting and screening of care must take place as in larger facilities. Where a case is recognized as failing to meet standards, the small medical staff or department should refer it to an appropriate specialist who is not on the medical staff or in the community. If this objective, disinterested review, confirms that the standard of care has not been met, the small medical staff has a measure of safety in taking corrective action. It is not absolute because the assertion can be made that the selection of the outside reviewer was itself biased toward a predetermined judgment. Scrupulous attention to fairness and referral to several reviewers will help to reduce further the risk of challenge. Physicians who serve on a hearing panel and the hearing officer should also be carefully screened for evidence of bias, malice, or conflict of interest.

Challenge can be mitigated both in small and large settings if the physician is given an opportunity to change behavior and improve before the limitation or restriction is imposed. Most problems of physician performance can probably be managed this way.[15,16]

☐ *References*

1. Liset, J. R. Musick, Peeler and Garrett, Conducting the Hearing: Legal Requirements and Practical Solutions, presented as part of the American Bar Association Forum Committee on Health Law program, "Peer Review and the Law" (May 1986); program materials published by the ABA or available from the author, Los Angeles, CA.

2. Lohr, K. N. *Medicare: A Strategy for Quality Assurance.* Vol. 1, pp. 126–27. Washington, DC: Institute of Medicine, National Academy Press, 1990.

3. Joint Commission on Accreditation of Healthcare Organizations. *Accreditation Manual for Hospitals.* Oakbrook, IL: JCAHO, 1990.

4. Liset, J. R.

5. Health Care Quality Improvement Act of 1986, Pub L 99-660.

6. Patrick v. Burget, 846, U.S. 94 (1988).

7. Reviewing doctors and hospitals are immune from antitrust liability, 90 Daily Journal, DAR 2608.

8. Christensen, J. D. Peer review immunities applied in antitrust case. *Los Angeles County Medical Association Physician* 120:23–25, 1990.

9. *Immunity for Peer Review Participants in Hospitals.* Chicago: American Academy of Hospital Attorneys, American Hospital Association, 1990.

10. Darling v. Charleston Community Hospital, 33 Ill.2d 326, 211 2d 253 (1965).

11. Gonzalez v. Nork, No. 228566 (Superior Court, Cal. Sacramento County, Nov. 19, 1973).

12. Elam v. College Park, 132 Cal. App. 3d 232, modified 133 Cal.App.3d 94a (Ct App. 1982).

13. Joint Commission on Accreditation of Healthcare Organizations. *Accreditation Manual for Hospitals [published annually].*

14. Crane, M. How much do you risk when you review a colleague's work? *Medical Economics* 66(17):23–28, Sept. 4, 1989.

15. Eisenberg, J. M. Doctors' decisions and the cost of medical care. *Health Administration Press Perspectives.* Ann Arbor, MI: Health Administration Press, 1986.

16. Sheldon, A. *Managing Doctors.* Homewood, IL: Dow Jones-Irwin, 1986.

☐ Chapter 9

Motivating Effective Peer Review

Why does peer review work? What collection of social and political attributes will lead members of a medical staff to donate free time and risk personal and legal disapprobation in the judgment of their fellows? Are the rewards of behavior modification and restraint of errant physicians an end in themselves, or is there some grander goal that drives the process?

We know from the experience of the JCAHO that there is substantial variability in the sophistication and effectiveness of medical staffs.[1] Adherence to an accrediting standard is not sufficient to motivate effective peer review by the medical staff. Regulation is equally ineffective. Even though all states and the federal government have requirements for licensure and reimbursement that mandate effective and assertive peer review, the process still may be ineffective or nonexistent. Inspection and citation obviously can invoke an obedient response, but the resultant peer review and medical staff processes are likely to remain reluctant or diffident.

Yet there are medical staffs that have it all together. They have an internal cohesion that establishes a pattern of clinical and social behavior to which most of their members conform without obvious external constraint. Limitation, if deemed necessary, is applied in defense of the common standard, with the consensus of the group, including the physician who is limited as a result.

Consensus and a willingness to accept group standards are a function of the value that the individual receives from participation.[2] A physician who joins a medical staff that provides nothing in return except access to a hospital bed is not likely to make the necessary commitment. Where the medical staff meets the needs and expectations of the physician, membership will be worth more.[3] Conformity to and support of group process are more likely to follow.

Sometimes, a physician's willingness to accept medical staff standards can develop even if expectations are not met. A hospital that is the only game in town may thrive in the absence of peer review and medical staff standards. Similarly, some physicians will obey rules slavishly because of early training. A medical staff with a predominance of such physicians is likely to be a more orderly bunch.

Except for these extremes, it is necessary for the medical staff to meet the expectations of its individual members to achieve its purposes as a group. Even where the physician is employed by the group, more than money must be provided to achieve the level of commitment required for effective peer review.

□ Physician Expectations of the Medical Staff

What, then, are the expectations of a physician who joins a medical staff? In the course of interviewing approximately 200 applicants for medical staff membership in a community hospital, the author has identified eight basic expectations:

* Professional autonomy
* Control of quality
* Patient advocacy
* Peer reliability
* Fair processes
* Equal access
* Access to information
* Consistency of hospital services

These are not rank ordered; each may assume dominance depending on the issue at hand.

The thesis is simple. By meeting these eight expectations, the individual will perceive value in the group relationship. Value will lead to defense of group processes and standards, despite personal cost. For the group, then, understanding and meeting these expectations is its reason for being. The group must be aware of the expectations of its members in all actions it takes.

Professional Autonomy

The core value of the physician is his or her autonomy as a professional. It is the right to establish a relationship with a patient. That right is granted by law but is modified by circumstance, choice, and medical staff membership. Autonomy includes the physician's ability to decide where to practice as well as what specialty or service to provide. Autonomy extends to the decision regarding which patient to treat, the evaluation of that patient, and selection and application or prescription of the treatment. Autonomy includes the independent right to terminate treatment and order disposition of the patient.

Medical staff membership limits this autonomy at nearly every level. The novice physician is surprised by that limitation but ultimately comes to accept it, if it is evenly applied. Thus a new member learns that the privilege of specialization carries with it training and practice requirements imposed by the staff. As well, with specialization comes restriction of privileges within the scope of the specialty. The unique patient–physician relationship is also limited by medical staff standards, utilization management, quality review, and discharge planning functions. Practice guidelines will further limit physician autonomy.[4]

Despite these constraints, the individual physician expects that the medical staff will recognize the value of autonomy and respect it and defend it wherever possible. The staff acknowledges the inherent tension between professional autonomy and peer review and allows for individual judgment. Where the medical staff undergoes restructuring to service managed care plans, the unique one-on-one relationship between pat: ¬t and physician is retained. Where it is necessary to abridge that on¬ n-one relationship to service a particular contract, that abridgment will be held to a minimum within the bounds of professional standards of care.

Control of Quality

The novice physician takes pride in a thorough grounding in professional standards. Based on the hubris of freshly concluded training, there is the expectation that he or she is the sole determinant of quality in the care of the individual patient. Early culture shock comes with the recognition that, on completion, the standards of the residency are replaced by the standards of the hospital medical staff. This realization is mitigated by the knowledge that physicians still determine the quality parameters. As a member of the medical staff, the novice has the opportunity to participate in that development.

The new physician is entitled to expect that the medical staff will have in place an effective program for the monitoring of quality. Integral to that program are objective measurable criteria and articulated performance and outcome standards. The program is supported by a group willingness to confront the failure of its individual members to measure up. Some groups, unwilling to identify substandard care or to insist on its upgrading, are misguided in their permissiveness. They deprive the individual of the growth and stimulation that come out of monitored adherence to high, articulated standards. The new physician is best advised to avoid joining a medical staff that offers "a hassle-free environment where you can do your own thing." This is an invitation to professional failure.

Patient Advocacy

The physician remains the advocate for the patient. Although other professionals claim a similar role—even the hospital finance officer carries the mantle during contract negotiations—the physician has the unique responsibility for determining the special patient needs and managing the system so they are met. The medical staff must recognize that role and support it when it is legitimately exercised in the pursuit of high-quality care.

On the other hand, the individual physician is limited by that medical staff support. Orders for the care of a specific patient must conform to general guidelines of appropriate care. Where the patient's needs transcend the level of care usually provided, the medical staff provides a group voice that is more likely to be effective in achieving the desired enhancement. Further, the joining together of the medical staff with the administration or the governing body provides an organized approach to patient advocacy. The medical staff and governing body working together are more effective in advocating the needs of their patients to outside agencies and regulators. The individual physician is entitled to expect the medical staff to provide this effective way of amplifying his or her individual voice.

Peer Reliability

The individual medical staff member expects that the other physicians in the hospital are at least on the same level professionally. For example, if the new physician consults a peer, there is reasonable likelihood of assistance and support. If the new member is asked to see a patient in consultation, it is expected that the patient has not been so badly managed as to represent an invitation for the physician to be included in a malpractice suit.[5] This minimum level of peer reliability provides a sense of security to the novice physician, leading to a sense of esprit and confidence in the group.

To achieve peer reliability, the medical staff must protect the quality and consistency of care by a program that provides:

- A high minimum-entry standard consistent with the needs of the hospital and the availability of physician resources
- A high performance standard
- A system for the objective measurement of performance against the standards

- A system for the aggregation of performance data into a physician profile on which is based the periodic evaluation and reassignment of clinical privileges
- A support system for failing peers, as determined by performance evaluation (failure that may be due to knowledge or technical deficiencies, problems of physical or mental health, or substance abuse)
- Corrective action leading to limitation or restriction of those peers judged to be unresponsive to supportive measures

Fair Processes

Given the right of the medical staff to take corrective action that can deprive the physician of civil and professional rights, as well as livelihood, there is an accompanying obligation for fair processes. These processes must apply to the initial request for privileges and membership. At the core is objective evaluation using explicit standards and peer review. Corrective actions are taken only with careful attention to procedural safeguards. Appeal rights are always available.

Where the individual physician understands the medical staff's review and corrective action processes, there is greater likelihood of acceptance, if not support. A reputation for explicit fairness enhances the authority of the medical staff action. A member limited by fairly applied corrective action of the medical staff has less chance of overturning that limitation by court action. Where the physicians perceive that the philosophic basis of peer action is scrupulous fairness, leading to higher standards, there is a greater willingness to participate in the review. Where there is a reasonable certainty that corrective action will withstand the hostile evaluation of courts and regulators, there is a sense of security that further enhances the willingness of physicians to be a party to it.

Equal Access

Fairness must extend beyond discipline to include those practice support elements that the hospital provides. The individual physician is entitled to expect a fair and explicit system for the allocation of beds for patients and time for procedures. A qualified surgeon may expect access to the operating room, its staff, and equipment; an intensivist or endoscopist has similar expectations. Where facilities are limited, there is a distribution system based on patient need, not on the political strength of the demanding physician.

Access must extend to the political structure of the medical staff. "One man, one vote" is the underlying principle for all who meet the minimum requirement of utilization and participation. That minimum must be reachable by the ordinary physician with an average practice using the hospital regularly but not necessarily exclusively. By that regular participation and utilization, the individual achieves the right to advance to positions of authority and control in the medical staff system. Ultimately, there is a fair and explicit way for the new physician to earn a right to share in the economic benefits of medical staff membership, such as access to referral panels, health plans, and managed care systems.

Access to Information

A special need of the individual physician is the knowledge and information available from the medical staff.[6] At a minimum, usually available even to casual users or emeritus physicians, is participation in the continuing medical education program of the medical staff. To be of value to the practicing physician, education should include socioeconomic issues and an analysis of the marketplace unique to the joint hospital–medical staff geographic franchise. Internally, the physician is entitled to current information about policies, procedures, rules, and services. More problematic is the point at which the new physician gains access to the planning functions of the medical staff and the hospital. For example, a physician who learns that his secondary hospital is planning to establish an imaging center across the street from his primary one will be tempted to share the information. Competitive and proprietary factors would tend to limit access to confidential data, yet even here there is often an advantage to be gained in promotion of medical staff cohesion. One cannot expect a physician to behave as a supportive member of a group if he or she is systematically excluded from the processes or results of some of its essential deliberations.

Consistency of Hospital Services

The individual physician expects that the hospital will respond accurately and consistently to a patient's identified needs. The role of the medical staff is to ensure that consistency by the explicit definition of professional requirements and the ongoing monitoring of institutional performance through the Quality Assurance Committee. A medical staff that is unable to assess in objective terms the hospital's performance is an ineffective advocate for patient and physician needs. The effective hospital–medical staff partnership arises out of the mutual acceptance of the service mission of both, merged in a cooperative and cost-effective way. Success can be ensured only by the explicit identification of goals and the objective analysis of performance.[7,8] Consistent quality performance leads to a strong community image that can withstand the occasional justified or unjustified adverse assault by regulators or media. A hospital whose public image does not have to be defended by its physicians is in a stronger position to induce their support. Effective peer review and the acceptance of group standards is inherent in that support.

☐ The Relation between Expectation and Motivation

The eight expectations mentioned in this chapter are more than a wish list; they represent essential components of medical staff function. They are capable of objective measurement and application. Systematically applied, they are a format for the organization of medical staff activity and a tool for evaluating its effectiveness.

The Medical Executive Committee usually operates in a reactive mode, dealing with varying skill and interest in those matters served to it at the monthly MEC dinner. Sometimes the fare is rich and meaty; at other times, it is spare and of little nutritional value. The result may be a feeling of pointlessness or futility of time and effort. Declining participation usually follows. One may use the expectations as an analytic tool for evaluating the needs of the medical staff at the beginning of each MEC year. A sample program might look like the following:

1. Professional autonomy
   - New projects to enhance private practice
     - Private office support systems
     - Development of physician-run ambulatory facilities
   - Protection of autonomy during review
     - Specialty-specific utilization criteria review and adoption
     - Support of internal and external reconsideration and appeal
2. Control of quality
   - Annual review of quality indicators for efficiency and effectiveness
   - Quarterly summary of departmental support and corrective action activities
   - Annual joint board–medical staff evaluation of hospital performance vis à vis the stated mission
3. Patient advocacy
   - Regular program for assessment of special service and equipment needs
   - Review of little-used services that may be obsolete
   - Medical Executive Committee assessment of departmental mechanisms for determining individual physician needs
   - Joint medical staff–hospital analyses of impact of major service shifts on efficiency and outcomes of care

4. Peer reliability
   - MEC oversight of departmental privilege criteria, for example, minimum requirement for training, performance, and current utilization
   - Analysis of departmental performance of specialty procedures according to objective performance indicators, including feedback data to individual participants comparing physician to group and physician to self, over time
5. Fair processes
   - Review of bylaws to ensure conformity with federal and state due process requirements
   - Training of active medical staff members in the art and science of fair peer review
   - Analysis of departmental and medical staff peer review and appeal experience
6. Equal access
   - Monitoring of access and scheduling conflicts as part of quality assurance program
   - Analysis of medical staff political activities to ensure broad participation and renewal of support
   - Incorporation of physician participation criteria in economic programs of medical staff
7. Access to information
   - A structured program of academic information, updating knowledge in common areas such as infection, surgical indications, new techniques, new diagnostic modalities, and the like
   - Departmental communication of quality assurance and peer review experience
   - Regular hospital market analysis
8. Consistency of hospital services
   - Annual assessment of community image, vis à vis regulators, customers, media
   - Monthly review by medical staff of patient complaint and risk management data
   - Objective analysis of effect of contract reimbursement on clinical services of departments
   - Annual assessment of hospital services in light of changing technology or professional standards

These examples, when organized according to the expectations of individual physicians, provide an inventory of group action oriented toward member needs. By recognizing an obligation to address the wants of physicians in these areas, the Medical Executive Committee sends a message that the group is concerned about the individual patient and the practitioner. A program that systematically addresses every category, as it sets its agenda at the beginning of the year or evaluates its accomplishments at the end, is less likely to be criticized for doing nothing for its individual members. By providing for individual needs explicitly and consistently, the medical staff gains support. From that support arises an internalized acceptance of the value of the group as a mediator and protector of the interests of the individual. Realization of that value leads to participation in the development and defense of the standards that characterize and strengthen the group. Broad achievement of that realization lies at the heart of the peer review process.[9] Legitimacy of peer review derives from that broad support. Absent that legitimacy there is no acceptance of authority; with that, order and quality are soon lost.

☐ *References*

1. Joint Commission on Accreditation of Healthcare Organizations. *Joint Commission Perspectives* 10(2):13, Mar./Apr. 1990.

2. Sheldon, A. *Managing Doctors.* Homewood, IL: Dow Jones-Irwin, 1986.

3. Lang, D. A. The medical staff is on your side. *Resident and Staff Physician* 33(13), Dec. 1987.

4. Lomas, J., and others. Do practice guidelines guide practice? *New England Journal of Medicine* 321(19):1306–11, Nov. 9, 1989.

5. Becker, H. S., and others. *Boys in White.* Chicago: University of Chicago Press, 1961.

6. Davis, W. M. Creating the nexus. *Physician Executive* 15(4):15, July–Aug. 1989.

7. Shortell, S. M. *Strategic Choices for America's Hospitals.* San Francisco: Jossey-Bass, 1990.

8. Coile, R. C., Jr. *The New Medicine.* Rockville, MD: Aspen Publishers, 1990.

9. Droste, T. Physicians want quality, support and governance role. *Medical Staff News* 17(12):6, Dec. 1988.

The Role of the Governing Board in the Motivation of Peer Review

The board cannot force the medical staff to do peer review. The willingness of physicians to perform peer review arises out of its perceived effectiveness in the defense of professional values. Simply put, if the medical staff has a clear image of its needs and goals, it will apply standards in the evaluation of patient care to achieve them. Peer review is a tool for the systematic identification of standards and a device for the control of physician performance within those standards.

The board cannot mandate professional standards, nor can it perform review on its own, as a substitute for physician review. True, in a situation of total breakdown, where the medical staff refuses to conduct review, the board could engage other physicians, outside the medical staff, to perform the study. Some bylaws permit boards to initiate corrective action. Even here, however, the medical staff sits in an appellate role ordinarily; it cannot be totally excluded by the board from the process.

The task of the board, then, is to foster the circumstances that lead to self-motivated peer review by physicians.[1] *Self-motivation* is defined as the willingness or drive of the individual medical staff members to take the time, do the work, and run the risks inherent in judging their colleagues. The board must actively support the medical staff by providing the tools, resources, personnel, and protections required.[2]

☐ Elements of a Board Program to Motivate Peer Review

If physicians value their hospital affiliation, they will support peer review to defend that affiliation. That support will be more than a willingness to participate in the review process. It will also be a willingness to submit to the constraints of medical staff review in the conduct of their own practice.

Physicians come to value a hospital that meets their needs and expectations. Reordering the eight expectations listed in chapter 9 to reflect the board's perspective, one can identify the following priorities for board attention:

1. *Consistency of hospital service.* The physician expects the hospital to provide a predictable level of care for his or her patients. That predictability should lead to public and professional perceptions of excellence, a powerful therapeutic adjuvant.[3] Nothing deters recovery more than the anxiety that the hospital or its medical staff is going to "mess things up again." A reputation for high-quality care makes the hospital marketable to a broad range of purchasers and is an unspoken defense against regulators and accrediting agencies.
2. *Fairness and equity in peer review and quality assurance.* Whereas the board ordinarily does not get into the details of the review of individual cases, unless they are appealed, the board must monitor the fairness and objectivity of the medical staff's programs for the review of care. Specific actions that the board can take to achieve this include:
   - Joint board–medical staff discussions of the processes of peer review
   - Joint agreement on the principles of fairness and due process
   - Negotiation of quality assurance and peer review data-base elements that comprise the measures of hospital and medical staff performance (see figure 10-1)
   - Annual analysis of peer review as a subject for joint board–medical staff retreats
   - Support of training for physicians and board members in medical staff processes
3. *Strong support for peer review in objective ways.* The board should:
   - Provide adequate personnel, hardware, and software to perform screening of patient care
   - Provide an adequate level of medical staff office services
   - Test adequacy by monitoring the timeliness of appointment, reappointment, and peer review
   - Consider professional medical administration, such as a medical director or paid chief of staff, to monitor and facilitate the peer review process. Note that the medical director is not a substitute for medical staff peer review, but is the agent of the board in motivating and evaluating physician review
   - Provide legal support the chief of staff can access to guide corrective action arising out of peer review

Figure 10-1.   Quality Scorecard

Elements in this scorecard provide a numerical display of the hospital's experience in matters of quality, risk, peer review, and medical staff function. Presentation of data on a quarterly and annual basis allows the board to be aware of performance levels and trends. If the same "scorecard" is used to communicate this information from the quality management function to the MEC and the clinical departments, then all levels are similarly informed. The common information base facilitates meaningful exchange and problem solving, free of the bias of ignorance or anecdote that sometimes dominates the exchange.

Mortality Rate
Medical _____
Elective surgery _____
Emergency surgical _____

Cesarean Section Rate
Total _____
Primary _____

Hospital-Acquired Infection Rate
Total _____
Clean surgical _____

Surgical Procedures
Appropriateness rate after peer review _____
Outcome _____

Medical Procedures
Appropriateness rate _____
Outcome _____

Drug Review
Current drugs studied _____
Appropriateness _____
Major reactions _____
Errors _____

Blood Review
Component use _____
Appropriateness _____
Major reactions _____

Medical Records
Incomplete charts—total _____
Incomplete charts—missing major report _____

Medical Staff
Applications pending _____
Reapplications pending _____
Rejections _____
Appeals _____

Peer Review (by Department)
Cases referred from QA _____
Cases justified _____
Cases received warning _____
Cases referred to MEC _____

Continued on next page

Figure 10-1. Continued

Liability Suits	_____
Patient Complaints	_____
Outside Agency Complaints	_____
Denials by	
PRO	_____
Medi-Cal	_____
Insurance companies	_____
Average Length of Stay by 10 Top DRGs—mean units of service per each	_____

- Provide an adequate level of insurance coverage to protect the physician. This coverage should be explicit for every physician engaged in review and should include protection for allegation of negligence, bias, malice, discrimination, and antitrust. Where possible by law, coverage should include defense of the case and payment of all awards. This is not always possible in antitrust or discrimination suits. If not, the physician should be so informed so that inadvertent personal exposure can be avoided.

4. *A positive program in support of the private practice of medicine.* Physicians perceive current restructuring of health care as a fundamental threat to autonomy. In the early 1980s, physicians turned to hospitals for support of traditional fee-for-service and individual practitioner arrangements. Although solo, fee-for-service medicine has not disappeared, physician concerns are now apt to be expressed in group terms. Access to contracts, centralized billing, purchasing, personnel or marketing services, and formal group practice arrangements are the more current issues discussed by physicians with their hospitals. Joint ventures have tended to fade as a business vehicle, as a consequence of a high failure rate and, more recently, federal limitations. At the same time there is recognition that the hospital and its core active medical staff share a geographic health care delivery franchise that must be recognized and included in any ultimate system redesign coming down the pike.

    The economic, legal, and personal risks of peer review in defense of the hospital's license are justified for the individual physician only if the hospital is seen as an honest partner in the economic struggle. It is not necessary for the board to try and buy physician support with marginally justified directorships or subsidized joint ventures. Hospitals in general no longer have the resources for these activities. Instead, the hospital and medical staff must come together in frequent and open dialogue, at a minimum involving leadership, to develop programs in the following areas:

- Support of physician autonomy; where practice is restructured by assigning responsibilities of the physician to a nurse or technician, the decision should be made by physicians and the results monitored as part of medical staff quality assurance
- Development of internal advocacy systems that solicit information in an organized way regarding patient and physician service needs
- Dedication of hospital resources to support physicians in private practice

5. *A program to strengthen the medical staff as a political decision-making body.* One of the frustrations of hospital leaders is the inability to be certain of the accuracy of information about medical staff opinions and attitudes. Expressions of medical staff public opinion are difficult to obtain at best. The typical medical staff pays inadequate attention to the soliciting and molding of opinion; consequently, when elected leaders speak they may speak only for themselves. Repeatedly, administrators or chiefs of staff are surprised when a carefully negotiated agreement blows up after the fact because it was based on an inadequate knowledge of the general medical staff attitude. Because of this phenomenon, there is an overemphasis on the need for consensus, the end result of which is minority rule, as one loud dissenter can thwart agreement.

   Peer review is an exercise in participatory democracy in that standards are developed in group deliberation. Authority arises from the adoption of medical staff bylaws that mandate processes and relationships that govern the peer review process. General medical staff support of peer review systems and actions is essential for success. Making the medical staff into an effective deliberative body requires positive action by the board. Some of the following steps may be helpful:

   - Develop communication tools to ensure wide dissemination of information regarding hospital and physician issues. Newsletters, general staff meetings, open forums, department meetings are all useful.
   - Allow ample time for review and comment and for medical staff quasi-legislative hearings to air discussion about contemplated major policy, service, or rule changes. These hearings work as follows. The Medical Executive Committee determines the need for a significant rule change, such as an increase in the utilization requirements to maintain attending physician status or the training required to be allowed certain specialty privileges. Passage by the medical staff is contingent on successful completion of the following steps:
     1. Promulgation of the proposed change to the medical staff
     2. Convening of a hearing open to any attending physician to present testimony regarding the issue
     3. Redebate by the MEC, incorporating the findings of the hearing

4. If the proposal passes, allowance of individual physicians to demand a formal judicial review hearing, with right of appeal to the governing body, to protest the new ruling because of personal adverse effects
Many bylaws provide for this mechanism. It is more orderly than waiting for the physician to break a rule and having to respond with punitive action.

- Monitor administrator performance to guard against a management style that fosters medical staff disorganization to facilitate manipulations of factions.
- Negotiate with the Medical Executive Committee regarding decision-making authority and responsibility. Items that require sign-off by both the medical staff and the board are presented in a timely way to allow real deliberation and decision making.

Figure 10-2 represents an allocation of medical staff and hospital responsibilities to consult and communicate, adapted from the *Report of the Joint Task Force on Dispute Resolution in Hospital–Medical Staff Relationships*, developed by the American Hospital Association and American Medical Association, though never formally adopted.[4] It makes the point that very few decisions are the exclusive province of either the board or the medical staff.

In reviewing how decisions are made in the hospital, the board and the medical staff should develop an explicit protocol that identifies the decisions that require informal consultation, those that require formal discussion and sign-off, and those that require formal joint development. The protocol will identify only a very small number of issues that the board or the medical staff can decide without each other.

☐ Study of 10 Hospitals with Good Medical Staff Relations

Shortell[5] made this point clearly in a recent report of a two-year study of 10 hospitals with good medical staff relations. The best organizations had strong and consistent direction. Administrators were in place for more than eight years in 7 of the 10 hospitals; in only one was the administrator present for less than three years. Managerial stability was also a factor. Strong, trained physicians, the product of well-developed leadership training programs, characterized the medical staffs. Having a medical director was found to be helpful; Shortell recommends at least a part-time director for hospitals with more than 200 beds.

The goal of strong hospital and physician leadership is to create a culture of collaboration and cooperation. Whereas some institutions are

Figure 10-2. Allocation of Decision-Making Responsibilities

Governing Board Makes Ultimate Decision			Neither May Solely Make Ultimate Decision	Medical Staff Makes Ultimate Decision		
No duty to consult → Singular	Informal consultation → Consultative	Formal consultation → Shared	Formal consultation → Joint	Formal consultation → Shared	Informal consultation → Consultative	No duty to consult → Singular
1. Corporate bylaws	1. Discontinuance of a service	1. Create new department	1. Rule on medical staff bylaws	1. Bioethics	1. Evaluate transfers	1. Medical policies
2. External relations	2. External relations, medical	2. Limit procedures	2. Select medico-administrative officers	2. Personnel use		2. Professional evaluation of quality of care
3. Monitoring of quality	3. Hospital services	3. Assign staff categories	3. Amend bylaws regarding new categories	3. Physician contracts, patient care functions		3. Application of utilization review criteria
4. Enforcement of sanctions	4. Marketing	4. Rule on access of non-MDs to hospital	4. Rule on closure of medical staff	4. Development of QA plan		
	5. Hospital diversification	5. Rule on impaired physicians	5. Rule on limited license practitioners	5. Corrective action		
	6. Outreach	6. Develop hospital rules/regulations	6. Rule on credentials			
	7. Mergers and acquisitions	7. Perform accreditation	• Institutional criteria			
	8. Corporate reorganization	8. Perform fiscal planning	• Professional criteria			
		9. Rule on contracts with third parties	7. Implement QA plan update			
		10. Rule on physician contracts, administrative	8. Enforce plan			
			9. Choose utilization review plan			
			10. Resolve impasses			

Source: Adapted from American Hospital Association and American Medical Association. *Report of the Joint Task Force on Dispute Resolution in Hospital–Medical Staff Relationships.* Chicago: AHA and AMA, 1985.

blessed with a long history of good medical staff relations, good relations were found even in facilities that had only recently discovered the advantages of working together. Open, consistent, and honest communication was the principal technique for generating mutual respect, if not mutual regard.

Some of the programs arising out of these close hospital–physician relationships included:

- A physician–hospital organization (PHO), outside the medical staff, to address economic, marketing, and practice support needs not met by the traditional medical staff organizations. These PHOs may be an independent practice association (IPA) or a joint venture or simply a vehicle for working toward an economic unity without formal integration.
- An effective quality assurance and peer review program that permits the evaluation of physician performance. A commitment to continuous quality improvement by the board, the medical staff, and the administration was an added plus. Open communication about quality issues was critical.
- Empowerment of physicians as partners in the hospital's planning and program development process. Allowing physicians to identify their own problems and encouraging them to solve them themselves, where possible, was found to be successful by some hospitals. Devotion of hospital resources and personnel to assist in the process was a key ingredient.

Some specific activities undertaken by the 10 hospitals in the group warrant consideration by all:

- A communication protocol to guide the administrative response to physician problems, elements of which include the prompt return of phone calls, number of days to address a problem, strategies for feedback, and management of nurse liaison problems
- One-on-one discussion with physicians where changes are of major consequence
- Physician liaison and practice enhancement programs that may include support of office personnel and functions
- Avoidance of destructive competition in ambulatory care
- Joint ventures to service managed care contracts
- Development of new, mutually supported inpatient services
- Development of hospital and medical staff mechanisms to monitor and manage change
- Training of young physicians to understand the techniques and goals of effective medical staff management

In summary, the study found that a successful and cooperative relationship between the medical staff and the hospital comes as a result of hard work, a commitment toward mutual support, and the presence of strong, consistent, and qualified leadership to carry it out.

☐ Conclusion

To reiterate, the expectations of physicians who join the medical staff provide the board with a vehicle for linking hospital actions to medical staff goals. It is not a "wish list" of goodies to be doled out in reward for patient admissions or as a bribe for not making trouble. Board policies and actions that identify physicians as valued members of the joint franchise in turn elicit a sense of pride and ownership in the hospital. Medical staff members speak of "our hospital" with commitment. The task of the board is to promote the concept of community that includes the medical staff. The medical staff will on its own motivation rise to defend that community. Peer review is the principal tool for that defense.

☐ *References*

1. McMahon, L. F., Jr., and others. The integrated inpatient management model. *Annals of Internal Medicine* 111(4):318–26, Aug. 15, 1989.
2. Grayson, M. A. Breaking the medical gridlock. *Hospitals* 63:32–37, Feb. 20, 1989.
3. Joint Commission on Accreditation of Healthcare Organizations. Proposed Principles of Organizational and Management Effectiveness for Health Care Organizations. Agenda for Change Update. Oakbrook, IL: JCAHO, Feb. 1989.
4. American Hospital Association and American Medical Association. *Report of the Joint Task Force on Dispute Resolution in Hospital–Medical Staff Relationships.* Chicago: AHA and AMA, 1985.
5. Shortell, S. M. Leadership key to hospital medical staff relations. *Medical Executive Committee Reporter,* Sept. 1990.

Chapter 11

New Directions in Peer Review

Peer review by the voluntary medical staff is not likely to persist in its current form. Despite the systems described in the preceding chapters, forces exist that will substantially modify the way in which physicians look at each other's work. The legal factors have already been outlined; in response to these, the risks and burdens of peer review have significantly increased. In addition, the advent of data collection outside the hospital by a variety of entities will place the medical staff on the defensive.[1] Outside monitoring agencies already know more about individual physician and aggregate medical staff performance than does the medical staff itself. Even now, the medical staff is forced to either discipline or defend its members in response to data collected by others outside the hospital.

These circumstances will necessitate a modification in how the medical staff reviews care and takes corrective action. An understanding of these changes is required to function effectively today as well as to prepare for the future.

☐ The End of Voluntarism

There is growing recognition that peer review is not a game for amateurs. Medical staffs turn to attorneys more and more to guide their committees every step of the way. Although such expensive guidance is laudatory, it sends the message that peer review has gone beyond the collegial to the legalistic. It has become time-consuming, risky, and threatening to the reviewer. As a consequence physicians, less willing to volunteer, are fueling a growing demand for payment for performing the review.

In its simplest form, payment is expected for direct hours spent in review. This is an extension of the payment practice sanctioned by the federal government in the Professional Standards Review Organization

(PSRO) program in the 1970s. Current demands, however, go beyond reimbursement for utilization review to encompass all physician review mandated or necessitated by a third-party payer. Included in this might be record analysis in response to insurance company, PRO, or licensure agency requests.[2] Some staffs do not pay for screening, only for definitive contested specialty review.

Indirect payment for peer review shows up in several ways:

- Payment for chief of staff or clinical department heads. In large hospitals, the chief may receive upwards of $50,000 for a 20 percent time commitment to oversee the medical staff's review functions.
- Assignment of peer review responsibilities to clinical department and specialty unit directors. Whereas in the 1970s the responsibility of a cardiology or pulmonary director was to enhance revenue by the promotion of utilization, many are now specifically charged with the restraint of inappropriate or unnecessary service through a process of concurrent review and control. They may assume the role of physician adviser described in chapter 4. Some medical staffs further empower the departmental director with authority to veto inappropriate orders for dangerous or costly services.
- Assignment of administrative medical directors or vice-presidents for medical or professional services.[3] An increasing number of hospitals have engaged physicians for these positions. Although the primary responsibility is to support the medical staff organization's peer review process, the medical director also functions from time to time as the ultimate physician adviser or peer reviewer. In the minds of some, this assumption of peer review authority by the medical director places standard setting and enforcement inappropriately in the hands of a hospital employee. The drive for efficiency in peer review seems to be overcoming this concern, but organized medicine is wary.

Some hospitals have created special internal review panels to hear formal peer review appeals. Physicians who participate are trained in the formal hearing process in advance of a specific case. Training may include bylaws, simple legal procedure, fairness principles, and antitrust issues. A sufficient number of physicians are then available to permit the chief of staff to select a hearing panel whose members have no conflict of interest. Although this system works best in the larger medical staff, the concept of acceptance of responsibility, in advance, to be rewarded by special training is applicable to even the smallest. Usually these physicians are not reimbursed for time spent in a hearing. Payment would expose them to the charge of conflict of interest; it would be seen as tilting judgment toward the hospital.

☐ External Peer Review

A growing number of organizations control physician practice outside the organized medical staff. Usually the organization has authority greater than that of the medical staff, including the ability to deny employment, payment, eligibility to participate in programs, autonomous professional behavior, even licensure. This transcendent capability to limit or punish the individual physician creates a unique problem for the medical staff. The latter is obliged to develop a strategy to respond to the physician sanctioned by an external body, despite exemplary performance within the hospital. On the basis of the action of the outside organization, the medical staff may impose its own restrictions on membership, privileges, or independent practice. The medical staff may also work in cooperation with the agency to modify physician behavior in anticipation of such limitations. The following sections provide examples of such organizations and their review functions.

Medical Groups and Health Plans

Many hospitals have contractual affiliations with groups of physicians. In the extreme form, as in the Kaiser system, membership in a single group, the Permanente Medical Group, is virtually a sine qua non for hospital medical staff membership. In other hospitals there may be several physician groups of significant size and organization making up the medical staff. Members may also be affiliated by means of an independent practice association (IPA) or a preferred provider organization (PPO). Medical staff membership is required for eligibility in these outside groups.

Each of these entities will have a review function that looks at both utilization and quality of care. Each entity is likely to have standards at least as stringent as those of the hospital staff. Well-developed ones will have a medical director who is responsible for coordination of the review program and for enforcing corrective action in more direct ways than might be available through the hospital medical staff fair hearing process. Communication between the hospital and the group medical staffs regarding physician performance may be an effective way of promoting compliance with quality and efficiency standards shared by both.

Consider the case of an obstetrician providing inpatient coverage of the patients of a health plan. The physician exhibits a pattern of missed deliveries and slow response to complications during labor. Discussion between the chief of obstetrics and the health plan medical director identifies that on nights and weekends the geographic area of coverage is too great for a single physician. The health plan is given the opportunity to improve its coverage as an alternative to the medical staff taking action against the individual physician.

Professional Review Organization

Review of Medicare patients by the professional review organization (PRO) is intended to identify patients who have been underserved or otherwise inappropriately treated. Physicians responsible for their care potentially can be denied the right to reimbursement for treatment of federally reimbursed patients. The details of the program are beyond the scope of this chapter but, of necessity, all medical staffs have become familiar with it. From the point of view of this limited discussion, it is important to point out that the medical staff has a special obligation to conduct its own review of any case identified as deficient by the PRO. Where quality or utilization issues are appropriately flagged by the PRO, the hospital medical staff has an independent need to consider its own corrective action. On the other hand, if the PRO is in error the organized medical staff should rise to its members' defense.

Health Insurance Companies

Many service plans, carriers, and self-insured companies have compiled substantial data bases regarding individual physician practices. Metropolitan Life Insurance Company and Blue Shield of California are two examples of leaders in this activity.

Patterns are emerging in insurance company data bases, indicating more efficient physicians or those with better outcomes. The Med-Par data base for Medicare patients has similar information. One expressed goal of these data bases is to identify the most cost-effective providers who would be the most preferred for contracting. The physician with the poorest efficiency and outcome numbers, on the other hand, is likely at some point to be excluded by the payer. These data are also used to trace fraudulent utilization and pricing practices.

Medical staff and hospital IPAs and health maintenance organizations (HMOs) are also tracking economic and outcome data. Still in its infancy, the process of relating cost to outcome will gradually improve to the point where physician productivity profiling will be possible at the hospital level.[4] Inevitably, medical staffs will be led to look beyond the outcome to the cost of getting there. In HMOs and IPAs particularly, the pressure will be to reward the more productive physician and to find a way of improving or removing the least productive one. Internal medical staff sanctions, as they follow, will heighten the tensions surrounding the peer review process.[5] They will underscore the passage from the scene of collegial review solely in the interest of improvement of patient care.

Professional Liability Carriers

Insurance carriers that provide liability coverage for physicians depend on the organized medical staff to determine clinical privileges. There is a presumption of coverage for care performed within the limits of the hospital privilege assignment. Possession of privileges by the physician is taken by the company as evidence of competence. On the other hand, regardless of the privileges held, the insurance carrier may refuse further coverage if it observes behavior that may be indicative of poor performance or incompetence in a case. The medical staff, then, may find itself in the difficult circumstance of noncoverage of one of its members. Where the medical staff has a mandatory coverage requirement, it may be obliged to take action against the physician's privileges, even if the questioned care did not occur in the hospital. Medical staffs now include questions about loss or limitation of liability coverage in their credentials evaluation. A history of such loss is a likely deterrent to medical staff acceptance of a new applicant.

External Review to Reduce Antitrust Risk

Much has been written about the need for fair peer review to avoid antitrust or anticompetitive motivation. *Patrick v. Burget*[6] is cited as a classic example of how failure to be sensitive to conflict-of-interest issues caused a medical staff peer review effort to ultimately fail. Regardless of the justification for review, bad procedure always undermines good content and motivation. The Health Care Quality Improvement Act (HCQIA) of 1986, which resulted from *Patrick v. Burget*, in effect set procedural standards to be followed that allow the medical staff to assert a defense of federal antitrust charges (see chapter 8 for a more in-depth discussion).

Despite HCQIA and similar protections in medical staff bylaws, physicians are seriously concerned about their personal economic risk as peer reviewers. Because an adverse decision arising out of review is likely to have a negative economic effect on the reviewed physician, the latter is likely to seek economic retribution against the reviewer. In small medical staffs particularly, it is difficult to refute the allegation that the elimination of one practitioner leads to some gain for those remaining. Even in a larger clinical department, declining aggregate patient loads could be cited as a support for the contention that one physician's loss is another's reward.

Besides HCQIA, added protections have been sought. One is a program recently adopted in Colorado where the initial evaluation is performed as usual by the organized medical staff.[7] Should the matter evolve to a formal hearing, the hearing body would be constituted as an agency of the state licensure board, so long as it conformed to certain legal process requirements. The formal hearing panel would thereby meet the requirement for exemption under the state action doctrine cited in *Patrick v. Burget*. That doctrine holds that no allegation of antitrust is possible where an entity is obliged by state supervision of its actions to be anti-competitive.

Contract Peer Review by Unaffiliated Physicians

Regardless of legal protections, some physicians find that they can no longer participate in peer review because of the potential economic threats. Others have seen entrepreneurial opportunity here to set up a panel of peer reviewers for hire. Typically, one or a group of physicians will advertise their availability to medical staffs or hospitals to review on demand. Services might include specialty review of a referred record, where an unbiased specialist may not otherwise be available. A more complete program would provide a hearing panel to hear a case. In either instance, the outside physicians would be granted temporary privileges on the staff for the sole purpose of providing the review and opinion. Because the outside physicians do not have a competing practice, no anticompetitive motivation could be attributed to their decisions. One such organization is the American Medical-Legal Foundation of Philadelphia.

☐ Who Determines the True Value of Medical Intervention?

Peer review at the medical staff level is based on what is perceived by practitioners as the community standard. Loosely set by conventional clinical practice, community standard is based on information in the clinical literature that supplements that obtained during training and experience.

A number of currents outside the organized medical staff may lead to judgments not held by the local group. As these judgments assume greater credibility, there is likely to be a lack of synchrony between the local peer review standard and that in the national literature. An example of this is the debate over coronary artery bypass surgery. Many medical staffs found the procedure to be effective in preserving function of the heart, while, at the same time, some national authorities were questioning its value. A similar debate exists about carotid endarterectomy.[8] Individual medical staff experience may lead to perceptions substantially at variance with national data.[9] In the resulting conflict, the national data are likely to dominate.

New technology is also perceived as more or less standard depending on local experience, availability, and willingness to pay for it. Computerized tomography is the classic case of a modality recognized as state-of-the-art by the professional long before payers and government would concede its value. Congress has just funded the first of what is likely to be a series of programs to achieve an agreement as to what constitutes effective care. Paul Elwood has called for a long-term national longitudinal study of patient outcomes as a means of developing further understanding of what works and what does not.[10]

Peer review bodies, then, at the medical staff level will find themselves working on an uncertain professional base (as well as the economic one described previously). The hospital medical staff is no longer the ultimate authority regarding clinical standards. It will be difficult to sanction a physician for omitting part of a workup, judged prudent by the medical staff, if subsequent outcome data might indicate that the omitted studies were not needed after all. For example, a current standard of practice indicates transurethral resection of the prostate for bladder obstruction. At the same time, other studies suggest increased risk and decreased utility for the procedure, at least under some circumstances.

Where the medical staff was in control of the peer review process, it could accommodate these kinds of shifting of professional sands. In the current era, however, where technology is changing daily and peer review actions are watched by state and federal licensure agencies, the medical staff may be unwilling or unable to take a firm line except in grossly inappropriate or incompetent care. Medical staffs must be absolutely certain about the scientific and professional basis for the actions they take.

Retrospective judgment of the courts that a decision was on insufficient or erroneous professional grounds is likely to lead to a further assertion that it was economically based. Thus, rejection of the action is followed by the threat of legal retribution for the "unscientific decision."

□ A Medical Staff Peer Review Strategy

Despite the foregoing concerns, the medical staff cannot escape its peer review obligations. In effect, the medical staff has no reason to exist outside of setting and promoting adherence to clinical standards. External review agencies have gained ascendancy over hospital medical staffs because the latter have been inconstant and ineffective in both developing and enforcing standards of practice. It serves no purpose to view the evolution of external agencies as antithetical to the role of the organized medical staff. Rather, that latter body, by state and federal law as well as individual hospital corporate bylaws, still has control of the decision making at the hospital level. Where that control is effectively and honestly exercised, it is not likely to be supplemented by outside authority.

The goal of individual hospital medical staffs and the entities that support them must be the promotion of peer review based on modern standards. For example, the efforts of the American Medical Association in conjunction with the Rand Corporation to develop practice parameters should be perceived as assisting the organized medical staff in setting local standards, rather than as undercutting the effort. Other specialty society guidelines are equally helpful.[11,12]

The American Society of Anesthesiologists, for example, has published a booklet, *Judging Clinical Competence,* which describes a system of clinical standards. On the basis of the work of Terry S. Vitez, M.D., the experience of Las Vegas anesthesiologists was collected to form the basis for judging performance. The system links clinical standards, quality assurance, performance evaluation, and privilege adjustment in a coherent way. Because the program is communitywide, it cuts across individual medical staff lines, creating an area standard both for patient care and medical staff peer review.[13] The program's use of strict numerical performance standards, however, may be too rigid in application.

Medical staffs should have a standards review function or committee that monitors change continuously. Educating physician reviewers in these changes is one way to ensure that decisions are not based on narrow or outdated concepts. Similarly, regular review of quality assurance screens to ensure that they represent current technology and standards is another way of guaranteeing that good information drives the peer review process.

Chapter 12 presents a system of peer review self-evaluation for the organized medical staff. It describes a series of elements associated with effective peer review. Regular assessment of medical staff activity using a scheme of this sort will be helpful in maintaining and promoting effective peer review.

Medical staffs must work actively to create an effective peer review process. This book has been an effort to identify the essential elements. The checklist in chapter 12 will be of further assistance in pinpointing opportunities for improvement. The list should be used as part of the annual review the medical staff conducts of its activities. That review may include readiness for accreditation and licensure surveys. Effective peer review requires more, however.

☐ *References*

1. Wennberg, J. E., and others. An assessment of prostatectomy for benign urinary tract obstruction. *Journal of the American Medical Association* 259(20):3027–30, May 27, 1988.

2. Larkin, H. What used to be staff duty is now an extra. *American Medical News,* May 25, 1990, p. 17.

3. Smaller hospitals looking to medical directors. *Medical Staff Leader* 18(6):1,8, June 1989.

4. Tierney, W. M., and others. The effect on test ordering of informing physicians of the charges for outpatient diagnostic tests. *New England Journal of Medicine* 322(21):1499–1504, May 24, 1990.

5. Goldman, L. Changing physicians' behavior. *New England Journal of Medicine* 322(21):1524–25, May 24, 1990.

6. Patrick v. Burget, 846, U.S. 94 (1988).

7. Professional Review of Health Care Providers, Colorado Senate Bill 261 amending Section 1, Title 12 Colorado Revised Statutes, 1985.

8. Winslow, C. M. The role of guidelines in achieving rational healthcare management. *The Internist* 31(5):14–16, May 1990.

9. Feussner, J. R., and Matchar, D. B. Diagnostic evaluation of the carotid arteries position paper, Health and Policy Committee, American College of Physicians. *Annals of Internal Medicine* 109(10):805–18, Nov. 15, 1988.

10. Curry, W. Outcomes management: new name for an old idea. *Physician Executive* 15(5):2, Sept.–Oct. 1989.

11. Getting it right: the making of practice guidelines. Theme issue. *Quality Review Bulletin* 16(2), Feb. 1990.

12. Guidelines for Development of Practice Guidelines, Report K, American Society of Internal Medicine, Report of the Board of Trustees to the 1989 House of Delegates.

13. *Judging Clinical Competence,* a booklet. American Society of Anesthesiologists, 1989, 515 Busse Highway, Park Ridge, IL 60068.

Evaluating Peer Review Readiness and Performance

The message of this book has been that an effective peer review program is the result of a deliberate process. It does not begin with the presentation ⸍ a chart to a physician for an opinion. Peer review can be effective onl, where there is a true peer group with shared values and goals. Achievement of this depends on a willingness of the individual to entrust his or her fate to the group because of the need to belong and some measure of faith in its processes. The medical staff leadership is responsible for the monitoring of those processes to ensure that they truly fulfill the goals of an effective peer review program. As peer review is the reason medical staffs need to exist, it is worth the effort of the leadership to implement a system for evaluating peer review readiness and performance.

Five general categories of indicators are suggested for self-evaluation: procedure, program, training, output, and threshold event. The following checklist elaborates on these categories. Using them annually to review medical staff structure and experience will help to identify potential areas for improvement in the peer review process. Consult the chapter references in parentheses for more details.

□ Medical Staff Procedure Indicators

1. Explicit standards for medical staff membership beyond licensure and practice in the hospital service area (see figure 12-1 for an example of screening criteria)
2. Interview of the applicant (chapter 3)
3. Proctoring concurrently at time of appointment, and, perhaps, prior to reappointment, granting of new privileges (chapter 3)

Figure 12-1. Screening Criteria to Be Given Special Weight in Reviewing Applications to the Medical Staff

- Board certification in major specialty and eligibility in subspecialty where appropriate; recertification where appropriate
- References by or personally verifiable by members of the active medical staff
- Successful completion of education and training in a program of known superiority
- Local practitioner of good reputation known to the medical staff
- Skills or attributes currently lacking in the center
- Office location and practice pattern indicating an enhanced ability to provide timely care of critical patients
- No adverse recommendation from any source
- Results of interviews with the medical director and/or senior representative of respective departments
- Academic appointment with current teaching activity
- Information from outside agencies

4. Explicit standards for privilege eligibility based on defined levels of skill, training, experience, and current utilization (see figures 12-2 and 12-3 for suggested components)
5. Concurrent screening of patient care employing an integrated approach that looks at utilization, service, quality, generic outcome, and patient satisfaction indicators (chapter 4)
6. Focused peer review or exception review to identify causes of deviations from standards of practice (chapter 5)
7. Graded corrective action guided by criteria based on severity of injury, degree of deviation from professional standards, and personal physician factors (chapter 7)

☐ Program Indicators

1. Motivation of peer review by a structured program to meet physician expectations (chapter 9)
2. Development of joint medical staff–hospital values regarding peer review, community service, commitment to quality, cost-effective service, and bioethics (figure 12-4)
3. Development of physician-performance profiles that track productivity, quality, utilization, peer review, and service
4. Development of departmental performance standards for comparison with individual performance (chapter 6)
5. Annual review of the medical staff screening indicators and practice standards to ensure relevancy to the current case mix and efficacy in identifying cases for review

6. Quarterly review of peer review and performance data by the Medical Executive Committee and the governing body (chapter 10, figure 10-1)

☐ Peer Review Training Indicators

1. Orientation of new physicians to the unique peer review systems and values of the medical staff

Figure 12-2. Standards for Privilege Eligibility

Minimum Training

Minimum Supervised Performance
  a. During training
  b. Proctoring

Current Use of Privilege

Likely Future Use

Acceptable Exercise
  Appropriateness
  Competence
  Outcome

Acceptable Volume

Figure 12-3. Standards for Privilege to Assist

Category I (most complex)
Assistant has same training as surgeon

  Examples: Pancreatectomy
           Total hip
           Radical hysterectomy
           Craniotomy

Category II (intermediate complexity)
Assistant has completed training in general surgery or equivalent experience

  Examples: Laminectomy
           Craniotomy
           Nephrectomy
           Gastrectomy

Category III (least complex)
Assistant has completed at least one year of general surgery training

  Examples: Appendectomy
           Cholecystectomy
           Compound fracture
           Herniorrhaphy

Figure 12-4. Bonding with Values

Stresses vital partnership

Identifies common values
   Life is sacred—futile care is not
   Quality care requires clear, respectful communication
   Informed consent and refusal are central patient rights
   Challenge peer performance
   Challenge hospital performance
   Recognize the vital role of nursing
   Universal access to adequate care

Shared commitment to common goals

Source: Reprinted, with permission, from Queen of the Valley Hospital, Napa, CA.

Author's Note: The joint value statement commits the hospital and the medical staff to common positions regarding the rights of patients, professionals, and the hospital. It is a unique guide to future joint decisions.

2. Annual presentation to the medical staff of aggregate peer review experience of prior year and new anticipated problems
3. Regular review of peer review matters in the medical staff newsletter
4. Training for the medical staff in the unique screening, chart review, and peer review systems of the hospital
5. Leadership training for top medical staff officers, focused on quality assurance and peer review
6. Specific instruction in the formal judicial review procedure for selected department members

☐ Peer Review Output Indicators

1. Data showing the results of screening of all significant clinical services, focused by experience of prior review to home in on problem areas
2. Data showing the number and disposition of cases identified for physician review
3. Data showing a mix of physician-specific, patient-specific verbal and written communication from the department to individual physicians
4. Referral of cases to the Medical Executive Committee for action
5. Judicial review hearings—reviewed by MEC and board, even if not appealed, to evaluate the process
6. Appeals of judicial review decisions to governing body
7. Court challenges of cases that have been in the peer review process

☐ Threshold Event Indicators

1. Cases identified de novo by lawsuit, PRO review, or licensure agency that on retrospective review by the medical staff lead to retroactive discipline after outside identification
2. Major iatrogenic injury not investigated by the medical staff
3. Hospital gossip or grumbling about failure of the medical staff to take corrective action in a "bad" case
4. Refusal of physicians to serve on screening committees
5. Refusal of physicians to serve on formal judicial hearing committees
6. Citation by Medicare or the JCAHO for failure to perform definitive case review or to take effective corrective action
7. Refusal of payer or health plan to contract with the medical staff because of poor quality
8. Published data indicative of poor outcomes unknown to the medical staff or uninvestigated after publication
9. Complaints of breach of fair process by a physician's attorney prior to a formal hearing
10. No judicial review hearings or unrequested privilege modifications in a five-year span

Whereas some of these indicators will be met by satisfying the accreditation standards of the JCAHO or meeting the Medicare "Conditions of Participation," in themselves those standards are insufficient to ensure support for the medical staff peer review process. Process, training, and output indicators go beyond minimum accreditation standards to address effectiveness, efficiency, and support of the peer review process. Threshold event indicators (and doubtless there are others) herald a major failure. Occurrence of a threshold event signals the need for a major inquiry and probable overhaul of the medical staff's peer review program.

Scenarios for Discussion and Self-Testing

Readers of this book should now have an understanding of and a system for peer review. That understanding may be tested by review of the six scenarios that follow. Each has a series of questions to assist analysis and promote discussion. Each illustrates the relationship among quality assurance, peer review, and privilege assignment. Issues related to corrective action are also highlighted. Scenarios such as these are useful as a point of departure for Medical Executive Committee meetings dealing with setting the standards for peer review corrective action and physician performance evaluation.

☐ Peer Review Scenario I

You are a member of the Judicial Review Panel hearing the appeal of Dr. John, whose charge reads that he has "violated the medical staff bylaws requiring provision of the highest quality of care." Specifics of the charge include:

a. A nosocomial infection rate of 5 percent for clean elective surgery
b. Two missed deliveries
c. Two patient complaints about high fees
d. A questioned hysterectomy that was identified retrospectively by a review agency

The narrative of the case shows that John was summarily suspended after missing the second delivery. The summary suspension was extended to 60 days following MEC review.

The medical staff presented the data and cases described in the charges. In mitigation, John cited the following:

1. The departmental infection rate was 4 percent.
2. He was unable to obtain the missed delivery rate for the department.
3. The risk manager had investigated the patient complaints and refused to share the data with the medical staff.
4. Other physicians had had cases denied by the review agency without further medical staff action.

Please answer the following questions:

1. Was the summary suspension appropriate?
2. Has the medical staff proven its case with respect to its charges?
3. What, if any, information is lacking?
4. Discuss the bylaws violation.

☐ Peer Review Scenario II

The Rhinoplasty Center of Excellence was a freestanding department of Plastic Ventures Hospital, Incorporated. Its four members were all highly trained surgeons who prided themselves on their ability to make curved noses straight or upturning. They were independent of each other and highly competitive.

Ethmoid, the newest member of the department, received a memo informing him that a case he had seen in the emergency room was coming to peer review. The reason was not given and, worse, medical records could not produce the chart for him prior to the meeting.

Committee review took place as scheduled, with Ethmoid present. Conclusions were:

1. Based on a postreduction photograph in the emergency room, the immediate management was found below standard because the nares were of unequal size and facial symmetry was not restored.
2. During the patient's follow-up visit to the office of another committee member three weeks later, the nose was described as unacceptably deformed, and reoperation was scheduled by that member.
3. A postreoperation film showed satisfactory reduction.

The committee found the care to be substandard and referred the matter to the department. When the department met, Ethmoid was excused from attending. He was judged to be unfit for dealing with nasal trauma and was dropped from the ER backup rotation, leaving the other three department members to share the rotation.

Please answer the following questions:

1. Was the peer review committee acting properly in reviewing the case?
2. Were the data adequate to establish substandard care?
3. Was the departmental action appropriate?

☐ Peer Review Scenario III

A 72-year-old surgeon is referred from QA because of a 20 percent wound dehiscence rate. On his next case, before any additional review, he removes a normal gallbladder. Called to the Surgical Peer Review Committee to discuss these observations, he resigns from the medical staff rather than appear.

Two years elapse during which he operates at another hospital. He then requests a reinstatement of his privileges. Your surgical census is low.

Please answer the following questions:

1. What are the pros and cons of taking him back?
2. If you refuse to accept him, what is the basis? Do you need other data?
3. If you accept him, what privileges would you grant him? How would you protect the hospital from an allegation of negligence on the part of the governing body for failure to ensure patient safety through effective peer review?
4. Should he be reported to the National Practitioner Data Bank? If so, when and for what reason?

☐ Peer Review Scenario IV

The finance officer informs you as chief of staff that a physician with an average census of 20 Medicare and Medicaid patients is costing the hospital money. The physician, whose patients are all outliers, orders lab tests and X rays with great frequency and all of the cases have five or more consultants. She is known as a cautious but good physician by colleagues, but there have been several concurrent Medicaid denials, after which she still refused to discharge the patient. There's no prior disciplinary action for any cause. This physician has not changed practice habits despite a detailed discussion with the UR chairman about prospective reimbursement. The bylaws provide no requirement for cost-effective or efficient care.

Please answer the following questions:

1. Can you suspend her privileges or discipline her for any of the above?
2. Assuming the Medical Executive Committee was in agreement, what rules would you consider to rectify this situation?
3. Can you think of a strategy that does not drive the physician away while the medical staff changes her habits?

☐ Peer Review Scenario V

A wave of excitement washed over the Credentials Committee as it voted unanimously to accept the application of Professor Cutter. Albert J. Cutter, author of "Memoirs of the Limbic System" and developer of the "House Officers' System for Precise Neurosurgical Diagnosis," was leaving academia to join the staff of "our" hospital. Little Greenbelt Memorial, with its 60 beds, could now look to joining the big leagues. Visions of expansion of critical care danced before the administrator's eyes, and the several internists with latent intensive care skills envisioned yards and yards of pulmonary flotation catheters wedging up to the capillary opening.

The application file, barely examined by the committee, contained evidence of Dr. Cutter's academic appointment, a lengthy curriculum vitae filled with speeches, panels, and profoundly important basic scientific articles. References spoke glowingly of the physician's value as a teacher. His privilege card, requesting full neurosurgical privileges, had been signed by the chief of staff with a proud flourish. Imagine, stereotactic surgery at Little Greenbelt.

There had been one dissenting voice at the meeting. The neurologist who raised certain questions was shouted down for lack of vision and anticompetitive spirit. His minority report, which listed the following, was nearly torn up:

1. Cutter entered medical school in 1954; graduated 1960.
2. The years 1957 and 1959 were attributed to research, not otherwise specified.
3. In 1960–61, Postgraduate Year 1 (PGY1), neurosurgery at Elsewhere County Hospital in Big City.
4. In 1961–63, PGY2-3 at Elsewhere VA.
5. In 1963–67, in a neurosurgical fellowship at Overseas Institute.
6. In 1967–77, director of neurosurgery at Overseas.
7. In 1979–87, professor of neurosurgical studies at State College Hospital.

The enthusiasm of the Credentials Committee carried over to the governing board, which endorsed the privileges. Little Greenbelt had its neurosurgeon. Cutter lost no time. Conferring quickly with the anesthesia staff, recruiting the local general surgeon to assist, he began neurosurgical practice. His slow, meticulous style was taken as a sign of care. He needed no peers to proctor him; his fans knew his skills. To Dr. Cutter's credit, he performed several lumbar laminectomies with apparent success. Discharge of the patients on potent oral opiates was taken as a sad commentary on modern utilization review, which obligated early discharge. Cutter began to speak expansively and rapidly about his plans to create a neurosurgical institute to garner all of the work in the two rural counties around Little Greenbelt. The first planning meeting, in which Cutter spoke without interruption for two hours, came to an abrupt end when the director of nurses rushed in to report that her secretary had collapsed.

On examination, the secretary was in a coma. The neurologist said she had a cerebral hemorrhage. Cutter, over protests, performed a carotid angiogram and then, identifying a leaking aneurysm at the base of the brain, elected immediate emergency surgery. Exposure of the bleeding site was virtually impossible, but Cutter pushed on. After the administration of four units of blood (including one unmatched) during surgery, the patient's blood pressure bottomed and she suffered a cardiac arrest; resuscitation failed.

Cutter talked loudly and incessantly about the incompetence of everyone around him. He called for an investigation, which was led by the neurologist who had filed the minority credential report. The neurologist also had objected to the surgery. The neurologist concluded:

1. Cutter should never have operated under the clinical circumstances.
2. Cutter had privileges beyond his skills.
3. Cutter had dangerous delusions of grandeur and may be manic.
4. Cutter should be dismissed from the staff summarily.

The medical staff upheld summary suspension recommended by the neurologist. Cutter sued everyone in sight in state and federal court, asserting anticompetitive bias, malice, and extreme prejudice.

Please answer the following questions:

1. Were there any clues in the credential file to suggest that Cutter might have problems?
2. Was the hospital guilty of self-deception in accepting Cutter? In what way?
3. Was anything missing from the evaluation of Cutter's current neurosurgical skills?
4. Did Cutter show any evidence of impaired judgment?
5. Was it appropriate for the neurologist to lead the investigation?
6. Was the recommendation of summary suspension warranted?

7. Was Cutter justified in suing?
8. List five ways to avoid the "Cutter type" lawsuit as an aftermath of peer review.

☐ Peer Review Scenario VI

The administrator sat, pale and shaken, at his desk. His ear still pained from the phone call from the chairman of the board who had stridently read the newspaper account word for word. The reading was punctuated by, "How could Medicare say our care is of poor quality?" and "Didn't you have some way of ensuring that the physicians were qualified?" Not that the account contained erroneous information. The administrator's agony came from publication of the problem before he had received official notification.

The facts in the case were these:

1. The JCAHO in its regular triennial survey had identified significant deficiencies in monitoring and evaluation. Anesthesia did not have a peer review system. Surgical case review was limited to comparing the pathologist's diagnosis with the surgeon's, postoperatively. Case review, when performed, was recorded as a recitation of clinical facts with no conclusion and no corrective action. Reappointments were conducted every two years in two batches of 500 physicians each.
2. Medicare, having received word of the adverse JCAHO survey, performed its own validation survey and determined that the governing body was deficient in ensuring medical staff surveillance of quality. In addition to the JCAHO findings, the public health physician doing the Medicare review found three cases in which significant injury had occurred with little or no medical staff evaluation. One case had received a negative quality appraisal by the PRO.
3. The state entity that monitors hospital licensure was notified, and a statement of contingencies was sent regarding the three cases. A request for corrective action was included.
4. The administrator had filed the necessary corrective action plan.
5. The newspaper account came from unspecified officials in licensure whose policy it was to publicize such problems as an added inducement to correction of hospital problems.

As a consequence of the publicity, the administrator's corrective action plan was reviewed by both the board and the Medical Executive Committee. The administrator had acknowledged the failure of the peer review process with respect to the identified cases and the process problems identified by the JCAHO. Corrective action was promised within 90 days.

Hard questions about corrective action brought out the following:

1. The quality assurance coordinator was unable to provide aggregate performance data because she was the only department member and had only a word processor to assist her.
2. Attendance at department and peer review meetings was down. A number had been canceled.
3. Charts were flagged by a record room clerk after discharge.
4. There were no medical staff criteria for appropriateness of invasive procedures.
5. Physicians reviewed records only during the infrequent committee meetings.
6. The Medical Executive Committee and the administrator were in a "state of war" over the failure of the former to perform adequate peer review and the latter to provide consistent high-quality service.

Please discuss the following questions:

1. How have the hospital and the physician been adversely affected by the events?
2. Where does culpability for the situation lie? Board? Administration? Medical Executive Committee? Medical staff? Overzealous regulators?
3. List three goals (beyond getting the regulators off the hospital's back) to rectify the situation.
4. Outline a strategy to achieve the goals.
5. In your opinion, in the coming years is the hospital more or less apt to experience this event again?